Nutrition in Critical Illness

Editors

MIRANDA K. KELLY
JODY COLLINS

CRITICAL CARE NURSING CLINICS OF NORTH AMERICA

www.ccnursing.theclinics.com

Consulting Editor
JAN FOSTER

June 2014 • Volume 26 • Number 2

ELSEVIER

1600 John F. Kennedy Boulevard • Suite 1800 • Philadelphia, Pennsylvania, 19103-2899

http://www.theclinics.com

CRITICAL CARE NURSING CLINICS OF NORTH AMERICA Volume 26, Number 2
June 2014 ISSN 0899-5885, ISBN-13: 978-0-323-29918-3

Editor: Kerry Holland
Developmental Editor: Stephanie Carter

Critical Care Nursing Clinics of North America (ISSN 0899-5885) is published quarterly by Elsevier Inc., 360 Park Avenue South, New York, NY 10010-1710. Months of issue are March, June, September, and December. Business and Editorial Offices: 1600 John F. Kennedy Blvd., Suite 1800, Philadelphia, PA 19103-2899. Periodicals postage paid at New York, NY and additional mailing offices. Subscription prices are $150.00 per year for US individuals, $328.00 per year for US institutions, $80.00 per year for US students and residents, $200.00 per year for Canadian individuals, $412.00 per year for Canadian institutions, $230.00 per year for international individuals, $412.00 per year for international institutions and $115.00 per year for Canadian and international students/residents. To receive student/resident rate, orders must be accompanied by name of affiliated institution, data of term, and the *signature* of program/residency coordinator on institution letterhead. Orders will be billed at individual rate until proof of status is received. Foreign air speed delivery is included in all *Clinics* subscription prices. All prices are subject to change without notice. **POSTMASTER:** Send address changes to *Critical Care Nursing Clinics of North America*, Elsevier Health Sciences Division, Subscription Customer Service, 3251 Riverport Lane, Maryland Heights, MO 63043. **Customer Service: 1-800-654-2452 (US and Canada); 314-447-8871 (outside US and Canada). Fax: 314-447-8029. E-mail: JournalsCustomerService-usa@elsevier.com (for print support) and JournalsOnlineSupport-usa@elsevier.com (for online support).**

Reprints. For copies of 100 or more of articles in this publication, please contact the Commercial Reprints Department, Elsevier Inc., 360 Park Avenue South, New York, New York, 10010-1710; Tel.: 212-633-3874, Fax: 212-633-3820, and E-mail: reprints@elsevier.com.

Critical Care Nursing Clinics of North America is covered in *MEDLINE/PubMed (Index Medicus), International Nursing Index, Nursing Citation Index, Cumulative Index to Nursing and Allied Health Literature,* and *RNdex Top 100.*

Contributors

CONSULTING EDITOR

JAN FOSTER, PhD, RN, CNS
College of Nursing, Texas Woman's University, Houston, Texas

EDITORS

MIRANDA K. KELLY, DNP, APRN
Critical Care Nurse Practitioner, Critical Care Units, Memorial Hermann The Woodlands Hospital, The Woodlands; Instructor of Clinical Nursing, University of Texas-Health Science Center, Houston, Texas

JODY COLLINS, MSN, RN
Director, Clinical Projects and Magnet Program, Memorial Hermann The Woodlands Hospital, The Woodlands, Texas

AUTHORS

GORDANA BOSNIC, MS, RD, LDN
Clinical Dietitian, Food and Nutrition Department, Winchester Hospital, Winchester, Massachusetts

JODY COLLINS, MSN, RN
Director, Clinical Projects and Magnet Program, Memorial Hermann The Woodlands Hospital, The Woodlands, Texas

MICHAEL DINAPOLI, PharmD
PGY2 Critical Care Pharmacy Resident, Department of Pharmacy, UMass Memorial Medical Center, Worcester, Massachusetts

GEORGIA DITZENBERGER, NNP-BC, PhD
Assistant Professor, Neonatology Division, CHS Department of Pediatrics, UW-Madison School of Medicine and Public Health; Director, UWMF NICU Advanced Practice Provider Team; Manager, Neonatal Simulation Education, Neonatal Simulation Education Center, Meriter Hospital, Inc; Adjunct Faculty, UW-Madison School of Nursing Madison, Wisconsin

MIRANDA K. KELLY, DNP, APRN
Critical Care Nurse Practitioner, Critical Care Units, Memorial Hermann The Woodlands Hospital, The Woodlands; Instructor of Clinical Nursing, University of Texas-Health Science Center, Houston, Texas

MELISSA A. MILLER, PharmD, BCPS
Clinical/Operations Pharmacy Manager - Emergency Department, Department of Pharmacy, New York Presbyterian Hospital, Columbia University Medical Center, New York, New York

MARTHE J. MOSELEY, PhD, RN, MSN, CCNS
Associate Director Clinical Practice, Office of Nursing Services, Veterans Healthcare Administration, Washington, DC; Professor, Rocky Mountain University of Health Professions, Provo, Utah

JAN POWERS, PhD, RN, CCRN, CCNS, CNRN, FCCM
St. Vincent Hospital, Indianapolis, Indiana

BRITNEY ROSS, PharmD, BCPS
Clinical Pharmacy Specialist in Emergency Medicine, Department of Pharmacy, UMass Memorial Medical Center, Worcester, Massachusetts

KAREN SAMAAN, PharmD, BCNSP
St. Vincent Hospital, Indianapolis, Indiana

JUDY VERGER, RN, PhD, CRNP, CCRN
Director, Pediatric Acute Care Nurse Practitioner Program, Neonatal Nurse Practitioner Program, Pediatric and Neonatal Clinical Nurse Specialist Programs, School of Nursing, University of Pennsylvania; Pediatric Nurse Practitioner, Critical Care Children's Hospital of Philadelphia, Philadelphia, Pennsylvania

DINESH YOGARATNAM, PharmD, BCPS
Associate Professor, Department of Pharmacy Practice, Massachusetts College of Pharmacy and Health Sciences University, Worcester, Massachusetts

Contents

Nutritional support for premature infants in the neonatal intensive care unit setting is complex. Such infants have conditions unique to this period of the lifespan requiring specialized care management, both of which may impede the provision of adequate nutrition to support basal metabolic needs. Premature infants require optimum nutritional intake to support rapid growth during a time when they are not fully capable of tolerating it. This article reviews developmental anatomy, physiology, and the effect of premature delivery by systems; the challenges of providing adequate nutrition; and current evidence-based strategies to provide nutrition for premature infants during hospitalization.

Nutrition is an essential component of patient management in the pediatric intensive care unit (PICU). Poor nutrition status accompanies many childhood chronic illnesses. A thorough assessment of the critically ill child is required to inform the plan for nutrition support. Accurate and clinically relevant nutritional assessment, including growth measurements, provides important guidance. Indirect calorimetry provides the most accurate measurement of resting energy expenditure, but is too often unavailable in the PICU. To prevent inappropriate caloric intake, reassessment of the child's nutrition status is imperative. Enteral nutrition is the recommended route of intake. Human milk is preferred for infants.

Chronic critical illness is a problem in the critical care environment. The ultimate goal in managing care for the chronically critically ill is liberation from mechanical ventilation, leading to improved survival and enhanced quality of life. Clinical practice guidelines are presented as a framework in providing care for this distinct patient population. Research studies supplement the recommendations to ensure best care guides critical care decisions using the best evidence in the context of patient values and clinical expertise.

Malnutrition has been identified as a cause for disease as well as a condition resulting from inflammation associated with acute or chronic disease.

Malnutrition is common in acute-care settings, occurring in 30% to 50% of hospitalized patients. Inflammation has been associated with malnutrition and malnutrition has been associated with compromised immune status, infection, and increased intensive care unit (ICU) and hospital lengths of stay. The ICU nurse is in the best position to advocate for appropriate nutritional therapies and facilitate the safe delivery of nutrition.

Nutrition and care considerations in the overweight and obese population within the critical care setting are multifaceted. Patients requiring critical care have specialized care management needs that often times challenge health care providers. When patients are obese, this further complicates the physiologic aspects of healing, thus creating challenges to meeting both the nutritional needs of the individual and hampering treatment. This article reviews the care considerations, physiology of bariatric patients, and challenges of providing safe and quality care, including current evidence-based practice strategies developed to provide optimal support for obese patients during hospitalization and within the critical care setting.

This article presents an overview of postoperative nutritional requirements and goals following bariatric surgery. It summarizes current diet progression and nutrient intake guidelines geared toward optimizing weight loss and maintaining adequate nutritional status, nutrient absorption, as well as hydration. The article further emphasizes the importance of postoperative follow-up with a bariatric multidisciplinary team for appropriate postoperative care, diet management, and nutrient deficiency screenings.

Enteral nutrition is an important aspect of caring for critically ill patients, yet delays in implementation of guidelines and recommendations occur. Bedside caregivers are in a key position to evaluate current practice and lead change to implement evidence-based practice guidelines. Interdisciplinary teams can use change models, such as Larrabee's, to provide guidance and support success of practice change projects.

Recent data support the use of nutritional agents for use as targeted medical therapy. This article reviews some of the pharmacologic roles that parenteral nutritional ingredients (selenium, lipid emulsion, insulin, and levocarnitine) can play in the setting of critical illness.

CRITICAL CARE NURSING CLINICS OF NORTH AMERICA

NOW AVAILABLE FOR YOUR iPhone and iPad

Preface

Nutrition in Critical Illness

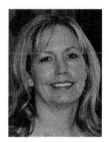 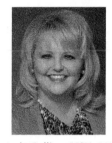

Miranda K. Kelly, DNP, APRN   Jody Collins, MSN, RN
Editors

Nutrition is an important aspect of care for any patient entering the hospital, but the patient admitted to the intensive care unit (ICU) is at an even higher risk for nutritional compromise. Nutrition affects all ages, from the neonate to the geriatric patient, and all patient populations. Evidence-based practice guidelines regarding appropriate nutritional support within the critical care setting are published. Yet, researchers continue to identify that despite published evidence, countless ICU patients continue to lack adequate and timely nutritional support on admission.[1,2]

Nutrition has long been an area of interest for us and is why we took this opportunity to be guest editors for this issue. It is important to us to share the latest information related to nutrition in critical care with more health care professionals so that all patients receive appropriate nutrition. Each of the authors in this issue promotes nutrition in their careers and individual practice areas, which brings knowledge from many different arenas throughout the nation. This issue discusses nutrition throughout the lifespan, special patient populations, implementation of guidelines, and how nutrition is being utilized as medical therapy.

The issue begins with an article by Ditzenberger that discusses nutritional support in premature infants, developmental anatomy and physiology, challenges, and evidence-based practice strategies in this population. The following article by Verger presents consideration for the pediatric patient populations in the ICU requiring nutritional support. The chronically critical ill patient is a growing population that often is admitted malnourished to the ICU. This patient population requires special care related to assessment, screening, and nutritional requirements, which Moseley highlights throughout her article. Powers and Samaan follow with their article with the purpose of discussing malnutrition in the ICU patient population. The authors elaborate on the importance of screening and assessment, delivery of nutritional support (enteral and parenteral), and issues related to nutrition. The malnourished patient is at a higher risk for complications related to nutrition. Therefore, the article also discusses the importance of nursing's role in relation to nutritional support as they are the ones providing care 24 hours a day.

Crit Care Nurs Clin N Am 26 (2014) ix–xi
http://dx.doi.org/10.1016/j.ccell.2014.02.006
0899-5885/14/$ – see front matter © 2014 Elsevier Inc. All rights reserved.

The obese patient population and patients undergoing bariatric surgery procedures are a prevailing population in the ICU. Health care providers may interpret a patient's weight as a sign of nutrition; in fact, obese patients are at risk for malnutrition also. Collins discusses considerations for the overweight and obese patient and specific nutritional requirements of these patients in the ICU. Due to growing obese populations, we have more patients that are undergoing bariatric procedures. These patients present with special considerations, not only immediately after their procedure but also for the rest of their life. There are different requirements for these patients in relation to the type of diet they consume, the administration of nutritional support, and complications, which Bosnic covers in depth in the following article.

The Institute of Medicine has reported that there is a 17-year delay in implementation of evidence-based practice guidelines into practice.[3] That being said, direct caregivers are instrumental in changing practice at the bedside. The Future of Nursing Leading Change, Advancing Health report recommends that nurses be full partners with physicians and other health care professionals to implement change in health care.[4] In the next article, Kelly discusses implementation strategies for enteral nutrition in the ICU utilizing multidisciplinary bedside caregivers as change agents. Nutrition is used not only to provide support to the patient in the ICU but also to treat medical conditions. We end our issue with an article by pharmacists Yogaratnam, Miller, Ross, and Dinapoli, who discuss utilization of selenium, lipid emulsion, insulin, and L-carnitine for the treatment of medical conditions.

We hope that you, the reader, will take the information included in this issue regarding nutrition in critical care and apply it to your practice. If not yet utilizing the evidence-based guidelines in your practice, ask why not. Health care practitioners can positively impact the care their patients are receiving by being engaged and continually learning. There are a number of resources available to guide implementation of nutrition support in all patient populations and we hope that you will be the change agent that your patients need.

Miranda K. Kelly, DNP, APRN
Memorial Hermann The Woodlands Hospital
9205 Pinecroft
The Woodlands, TX 77380, USA

Jody Collins, MSN, RN
Clinical Projects and Magnet Program
Memorial Hermann The Woodlands Hospital
9250 Pinecroft
The Woodlands, TX 77380, USA

E-mail addresses:
Mirandak12@sbcglobal.net (M.K. Kelly)
Jodyc42@gmail.com (J. Collins)

REFERENCES

1. Bourgault A, Ipe L, Weaver J, et al. Development of evidence-based guidelines and critical care nurses' knowledge of enteral feeding. Crit Care Nurse 2007;27: 17–29.
2. Cahill NE, Dhaliwal R, Day AG, et al. Nutrition therapy in the critical care setting: what is "best achievable" practice? An international multicenter observational study. Crit Care Med 2010;38(2):395–401.

3. Institute of Medicine. Crossing the quality chasm: a new health care system for the 21st century. Available at: http://iom.edu/Reports/2001/Crossing-the-Quality-Chasm-A-New-Health-System-for-the-21st-Century.aspx. Accessed August 15, 2013.
4. Institute of Medicine. The future of nursing leading change, advancing health. Available at: http://www.iom.edu/Reports/2010/The-Future-of-Nursing-Leading-Change-Advancing-Health.aspx. Accessed September 3, 2013.

Nutritional Support for Premature Infants in the Neonatal Intensive Care Unit

Georgia Ditzenberger, NNP-BC, PhD

KEYWORDS

- Nutrition • Premature infant • Protein • Extremely low birth weight (ELBW) infant
- Very low birth weight (VLBW) infant • Postnatal growth restriction

KEY POINTS

- Nutritional support for premature infants in the neonatal intensive care unit (NICU) is complex.
- Premature infants require optimum caloric and nutrient intake to support rapid growth and healing during a time when anatomically and functionally they are not fully capable of tolerating it.
- Providing nutritional support for premature infants in the NICU requires expert attention to detail and a working knowledge of the premature infant's developing anatomy and physiologic functions for all health care professionals involved in their care.

INTRODUCTION

Nutritional support for premature infants in the neonatal intensive care unit (NICU) setting is a complex issue. Premature infants requiring care have conditions unique to this period of the lifespan and require specialized care management. The condition and/or the specialized management may impede the provision of adequate nutrition to support basal metabolic needs and meet the needs for ongoing growth and development. Major advances in technology, pharmacology, and care management techniques during the past 50 years have supported the improved survival of all infants requiring NICU care, but especially premature infants. The surviving premature infants are affected by a myriad of conditions related to the level of immaturity, such as respiratory distress caused by surfactant deficiency and lung immaturity with the

Disclosure: The author has no conflict of interest or financial interests to disclose relating to the content of this article.
UWMF NICU Neonatal Advanced Practice Provider Team, Division of Neonatology, Department of Pediatrics, Neonatal Simulation Education Center, Meriter Hospital, Inc, UW-Madison School of Nursing, UW-Madison School of Medicine and Public Health, 4th Floor McConnell Hall, 202 South Park Street, Madison, WI 53715, USA
E-mail address: ditzeg@pediatrics.wisc.edu

potential for chronic lung disease, probability of complications related to patent ductus arteriosus, and a predilection for intraventricular hemorrhage caused by increased blood flow and vascular fragility of the germinal matrix between 24 and 34 weeks' gestation. Evidence indicates that nutritional support during this critical time plays a role in mediating the extent of the impact of these potential conditions affecting premature infants.[1-9]

Effect of Early Nutritional Support for Premature Infants

Premature infants require optimum caloric and nutritional intake to support rapid growth and healing during a time when anatomically and functionally they are not fully capable of tolerating it. Early nutrition during this phase of the lifespan has both immediate and far-reaching consequences for premature infants, from a role in mediating critical conditions during the initial hospitalization after birth, to later outcomes such as ongoing growth and attaining of nutritional milestones, likelihood of death, development of chronic diseases in adulthood, and neurodevelopment.[3,10,11]

Growth Restriction and Neurodevelopment

Compounding the effect of immaturity on organ anatomy and physiologic functioning, somatic, bone, and brain growth and development are at the highest velocity during the second and third trimester of gestation (when premature infants deliver) than during any other time of the lifespan; only growth during the first year of life comes close. Despite recent improvements in nutritional support for premature infants in the NICU, postnatal growth continues to be suboptimal, although there have been modest improvements in the severity of the issue. Numerous studies have shown that postnatal growth restriction is associated with small brain size and impaired neurocognitive development.[7-9,12-21] This association may be caused by the underlying inadequate nutritional support, which in turn is caused by the immaturity of the premature infant physiology and to the inadequate (but improving with research and evidence-based practices) nutritional products and management guidelines currently available to the NICU health care providers.[11] Providing nutritional support for premature infants in the NICU requires expert attention to detail and a working knowledge of the premature infant's developing anatomy and physiologic functions for all health care professionals involved in their care.

This article reviews developmental anatomy, physiology, and the effect of premature delivery by systems, the challenges of providing adequate nutrition, and current evidence-based strategies developed to provide optimal nutritional support for premature infants during hospitalization.

PREMATURE INFANTS: CLASSIFICATIONS AND DEFINITIONS
Premature Infant Categories by Birth Weight and Gestational Age

Premature infants are categorized by birth weight and gestational age; the lower the weight and gestational age, the more complex is the care required to provide support in the NICU. Very low birth weight (VLBW) infants, with average birth weight of greater than or equal to 1000 g but less than 1500 g, if appropriate for gestational age (AGA), are at greater than or equal to 28 weeks' but less than 34 weeks' gestation, and they have increasingly complex issues that compromise nutritional support in the first weeks of life. Extremely low birth weight (ELBW) infants, with average birth weight of less than 1000 g, if AGA, are less than 28 weeks' gestation, and are surviving in greater numbers with improved morbidity and mortality but have specific nutritional requirements and, by the time of discharge, may be growth restricted to the 10th percentile or less on standard growth charts.[1,20,22] In addition, premature infants who are small for gestational age (SGA) are associated with increased morbidity and mortality and pose increased challenges for nutritional support.[17]

Differentiation Between Gestational and Postnatal Maturation

Premature infants develop anatomically and physiologically on the same gestational maturation growth curve as their fetal counterparts. The organs of premature infants are mature to the point of delivery; that is, the gestational age at time of delivery determines the initial capabilities of physiologic systems to perform the tasks required to support extrauterine life. Maturation of many physiologic systems of premature infants is determined by postnatal age rather than gestational age in that the system matures more quickly in the extrauterine environment than in fetuses of corresponding gestational age. The postnatal maturation effect is limited to a functional level equivalent to term infants and to the limitations seen in term infants for each system.[23] To some extent, all physiologic systems are affected by postnatal maturation, with the exception of the brain, which is still in development phase during the third trimester.[23–25]

DEVELOPMENT OF ANATOMY AND PHYSIOLOGIC FUNCTION, AND EFFECT OF PREMATURE DELIVERY
Gastrointestinal Tract and Digestive System

Development of the gastrointestinal tract and digestive system
The pylorus, fundus, and gastric glands are formed by 14 weeks of gestation; the esophageal sphincter is present by 28 weeks of gestation. The gastrointestinal tract resembles that of a term infant by 20 weeks of gestation, and gradually lengthens throughout the remainder of gestation to approximately 250 to 300 cm by 37 to 40 weeks' gestation with gastric capacity of about 30 mL. By 28 weeks, there are the biochemical and physiologic capacities for limited digestion and absorption, with reduced production of gut digestive enzymes and growth factors compared with term infants.[23–25] Postnatal maturation effect increases absorption functions to near-term status over a period of weeks following initiation of enteral feeds.

Enteric Nervous System

The enteric nervous system is part of the autonomic nervous system, with the sympathetic and parasympathetic systems. Nerves with cell bodies within the gastrointestinal tract are a part of the enteric nervous system, which is more complex than either the sympathetic or parasympathetic systems. Intestinal motility, blood flow, mucosal secretion, and nutrient transport across the intestinal wall are mediated through the enteric nervous system.[26]

The primary formation of the enteric nervous system occurs at the time of neural tube folding into the primitive gut during the embryonic stage.[27] The newly formed gut is colonized with neural crest cells, which undergo an evolution process to reach the final forms and individual functional capacities of intrinsic primary afferent sensory neurons, interneurons, and motor neurons. These neurons perform both independently and interdependently to provide full gastrointestinal functioning. The enteric nervous system gradually matures according to gestational age, but is still immature until the bowel is stimulated with enteral nutrition. Full adultlike gastrointestinal functioning is thought not to occur until at least 1 to 2 years of life but may continue to mature through to adulthood.[24,26,27]

Gastric emptying

Gastric emptying is mediated by the enteric nervous system, which for premature infants causes transient feeding difficulties and potential for feeding limitations. Gastric motility is also limited by the immaturity of the enteric nervous system, which can cause interruption of forward peristalsis and may even show reverse peristalsis, and decreased muscle contractions of stomach and intestine.[26] The immaturity of physical functioning in the premature intestinal tract may cause delays in achieving full enteral feeding, especially in the first few weeks of life. The premature infant intestine seems to respond to postnatal exposure to nutrients, reflecting a postnatal maturation effect on absorption. However, motility and peristalsis seem to be governed by gestational maturation of the enteric nervous system.[24–26,28–32] The less mature the infant, the longer the time to motility improvement.[31,33,34] Small intestine motility is considerably less organized in VLBW infants compared with term infants, causing increased incidence of distention, feeding intolerance, and bacterial overgrowth. The bacterial overgrowth can lead to sepsis and/or necrotizing enterocolitis (NEC) caused by the increased permeability and fragility of the VLBW infant intestine and limited immune response.[26,31] NEC is associated especially in premature infants with low birth weight of lesser gestational age, causes prolonged and/or frequent interruptions in enteral feeding requiring prolonged parenteral nutrition, and the potential loss of intestine through surgical resection. If enough total intestinal length is removed or if significant small bowel is removed, a condition termed short bowel syndrome is the result.[35]

Feeding intolerance

Feeding intolerance is the inability or delayed ability to fully digest a volume of food between feedings, leaving gastric residuals and possibly abdominal distention as a result. Intolerance to feeding is a common occurrence for premature infants, especially when enteral feedings are first being introduced, primarily caused by the immaturity of intestinal motility of the premature infant.[36] Although some feeding intolerance as indicated by occasional increased gastric aspirate with or without abdominal distention is to be expected for premature infants because of the immaturity of the intestine, this type of reaction to feeds can be the harbinger of NEC and should not be taken lightly. For this reason, enteric feeding is often interrupted for periods of time for increased gastric aspirates and/or abdominal distention to determine whether the infant is experiencing just feeding intolerance or whether NEC is developing.

Necrotizing enterocolitis

Necrotizing enterocolitis is necrosis (death) of the intestinal wall, and is a severe disease affecting primarily the immature intestines of premature infants; SGA infants of all gestational ages are also at increased risk for NEC. Approximately 2% to 5% of premature infants have NEC, with an inverse proportion to gestational age: the less mature the gestation, the higher the incidence. About 90% of NEC occurs in premature infants and this incidence may be increasing because of increased survival of ELBW infants. In the late preterm and term newborns population, NEC is most often associated with prolonged rupture of membranes, low Apgar scores, chorioamnionitis, congenital heart disease, neural tube defects, and exchange transfusions.[37,38] Mortality is high for premature infants with NEC, ranging between 10% and 50%; in some cases of extreme NEC, especially for ELBW infants, survival is rare.[37]

Causes of NEC The cause of NEC is unknown, although there are many risk factors associated with the disorder, including a genetic predisposition, prematurity, postnatal age at time of initiation of feeding, aggressive enteral feeding, immature intestinal wall and immune barrier, bacterial overgrowth, and intestinal ischemia.[37,38] Overuse or prolonged use of antibiotics for premature infants has also been implicated as associated with an increased risk of developing NEC.[39–41]

Clinical presentation of NEC The clinical presentation of NEC often occurs quickly and includes abdominal distention and tenderness, occult or frank blood in stool, and shocklike presentation. Abdominal radiography depicts pneumatosis intestinalis, free air in the perineum, and sometimes portal venous air. Medical treatment, consisting of cessation of enteral feeding, antibiotics, and parenteral nutrition for a prolonged period, is initiated immediately. Surgical intervention with resection of the affected bowel may be necessary in addition to medical management when free air with or with out portal venous air is noted in the perineum or in cases of severe disease as manifested by shock, abdominal wall erythema, and/or bowel wall perforation.[38]

Short bowel syndrome
Short bowel syndrome (SBS) describes the inadequate functional length of intestine to support adequate acquisition of enteral nutrition and normal growth and development. Causes of infant SBS include surgical NEC with loss of necrotic bowel; volvulus, malrotation or atresia, with surgical resection of the affected bowel; gastroschisis, with potential for either or both surgical resection or loss of function of the affected bowel; and cystic fibrosis with intestinal malfunctioning.[42] The most important loss of intestinal length is that of the small bowel, where most of the nutrient absorption occurs; the colon's primary absorption function is for water and electrolytes and has less overall effect on the ability to eventually tolerate enteral feeds. There is a secondary effect of disease process in addition to bowel length loss that is a combination of both dysfunctional absorption and abnormal peristalsis of the remaining bowel, which further complicates effective absorption of enteral nutrients.[35,42] The presence or absence of the ileocecal valve is often used as a favorable sign for eventual success in enteral feeding for an infant with SBS. The presence of the valve may not be the sole reason for improved success in eventual enteral nutrition; it may be more likely that the remaining ileum attached to the valve promotes improved nutrient absorption.[35]

Renal System

Development of the renal system
Preterm delivery is associated with the interruption of attaining the full number of nephrons and with the development of the vascularization of the kidneys. Full adult compliment of nephrons is not completed until 34 to 35 weeks' gestation.[17,43] Nephrons are not of full length or functional status until past term for all infants, indicating some gestational maturation effect. Decreased glomerular filtration rate, altered tubular reabsorption and/or elimination, and decreased concentrating function further limits the premature kidneys' ability to perform adequate filtration and elimination of waste products and fluids within the first days to weeks of life.[23,44] Creatinine clearance and sodium retention improve gradually over the first 21 to 52 days of life, paralleling improved renal perfusion, stabilizing blood pressure control, and improved urine output, indicating postnatal maturation effect, but is still limited by the physical absence of the full complement of nephrons.[43,45,46] Adverse events causing insult to the kidneys that may further reduce adequate functioning include thrombi from umbilical arterial catheters, venous obstruction from indwelling umbilical venous catheters, overwhelming sepsis, or complications from patent ductus arteriosus or prolonged hypoperfusion.[23,45–47] Even without further insult to the renal system, premature infants are more likely to develop hypertension, endothelial dysfunction, and

proteinuria than full-term infants.[43] SGA infants have a higher risk for renal compromise than AGA infants, which increases the risks of complications, and special considerations need to be taken for fluids, medications, and advancing initial enteral intake.[48]

Primary functions of the renal system

Primary functions of the kidney include maintenance of fluid and electrolyte balance, acid-base balance, hemodynamic regulation, reabsorption of minerals and amino acids, and elimination of by-products and waste materials.[23,49] VLBW infants' renal systems at birth and in the first weeks of life provide variable function and become easily overwhelmed in the presence of excess fluid and solute load, and are easily affected by medications that require renal function to metabolize and/or eliminate by-products, or have an effect on renal blood flow.[23,50] Premature infants are at increased risk for developing electrolyte deficits, particularly of sodium and chloride, because of the immaturity of the glomerular reticulum and relative inability to resorb electrolytes and bicarbonate effectively during the initial period off peripheral nutrition/fluids/electrolyte solutions when on total enteral intake.[23,43,51] Renal function of premature infants approaches that of term infants within the first 21 to 52 days of life provided there has been no further insult to the kidneys beyond the developmental restrictions.[23,44,49,52] However, term infant kidney function is still only 50% to 85% of adult capacity, and can still be overwhelmed in the face of sepsis, fluid overload, hyperosmotic solute overload, medications, and iatrogenic insults to the kidney.[23,50] Term infants are therefore also at increased risk for alterations in fluid and electrolyte balance, although these difficulties are primarily caused by functional capacity rather than structural deficits. Adult functional capacity, including the ability to concentrate urine and retain/eliminate electrolytes to support bodily needs; glomerular development; and nephron maturation are attained by around 2 years of life.[23]

CHALLENGES OF PROVIDING OPTIMAL NUTRITION IN THE NICU AND EVIDENCE-BASED STRATEGIES
Nutritional Needs of Premature Infants

Nutritional needs of premature infants differ from those of a fetus of similar gestational age, especially for protein. Protein requirements are greater to provide for ongoing promotion of growth and development. Evidence supports adjusting enteral protein to allow for growth as the infant matures, beginning with higher protein intake when less than 1000 g and in decreasing amounts with increasing weight and gestational age.[11,53,54] Early initiation of protein-containing fluids within 4 hours of birth is also supported by current evidence to promote positive nitrogen balance, or at least decrease the negative nitrogen balance that premature infants develop when not receiving adequate protein intake. For this reason, current guidelines support early initiation of solutions composed of D10W (dextrose 10% in water) and at least 2 g/k/d amino acids.[3,53,55,56] Blood glucose levels must be monitored while initiating parenteral nutrition (PN) or any dextrose infusions, especially for ELBW infants, who develop hyperglycemia quickly on even maintenance glucose infusions because of a combination of insulin resistance and relative insulin deficiency in premature infants. Increasing the glucose infusion rate gradually allows acclimation and improved insulin responses.[57]

PN

PN is a hypertonic solution of nutrients given intravenously. The solution contains carbohydrates, protein, fats, electrolytes, minerals, vitamins, and micronutrients to provide nutrition until enteral intake is established. The duration of PN infusion may be a few days, as in the case of an otherwise healthy VLBW infant with gradually increasing enteral intake, to months, as in the most profound cases of SBS.[23,58]

The most common carbohydrate used in infant PN is glucose (D-glucose, dextrose), which is the main energy substrate for body and brain cells. The amount of glucose that can safely be infused depends on the clinical condition and maturity of the premature infant. The current recommendation for the glucose intake for just-born premature infants is 4 to 6 mg/kg/min (7.5–8.4 g/kg/d). Concentration of glucose intake gradually increases to a maximum of 12 mg/kg/min (17 g/kg/d).[57,58]

There is limited research that substantiates the current recommendations for carbohydrate, other than some evidence that carbohydrate is more effective than fat in promoting nitrogen retention for premature infants. There are concerns for long-term effects of early high carbohydrate intakes, which support the restriction of glucose loads to less than or equal to 12 mg/kg/min to reduce disproportionate body composition with greater fat than lean body mass stores. As a result, recommendations for carbohydrate intakes for VLBW infants will remain theoretic, balanced between the limited evidence of benefit and the potential long-term effects, until more research provides supportive evidence to determine appropriate values.[30]

Protein in PN is administered using a crystalline amino acid mixture, such as TrophAmine (B. Braun Medical Inc) or Aminosyn (Abbott Laboratories). Fat is given in the form of isotonic 20% lipid emulsions with high caloric density and is begun within the first 2 to 3 days of life, gradually increased as tolerated. Current recommendations for established PN are listed in **Table 1**. Premature infants require consistent monitoring of urine and other bodily fluid output, electrolytes, and glucose while on PN to maintain normal blood levels as well as normal fluid balance. This monitoring may initially result in frequent changes in the PN concentration of nutrients.[23,58] Once the infant is on optimum PN and few changes are being made in the solution, laboratory monitoring may be reduced in frequency.

PN may be infused via a peripheral or central venous catheter. Glucose concentration is recommended not to exceed 12.5% when administered via peripheral venous catheter.[59] In addition, peripherally placed catheters are difficult to maintain for longer than a few days, because of the fragility of infant peripheral veins. Centrally placed venous catheters infuse into a larger vessel, enabling higher glucose concentrations in PN as well as increased longevity and stability.[23,58]

PN-related Cholestasis

Cholestasis in infants with prolonged PN infusion typically manifests with increased direct bilirubin that usually resolves after PN is discontinued when enteral intake is established. Concurrent sepsis, intestinal surgery, and prematurity are confounding factors; as such, the pathogenesis of PN-related cholestasis in infants remains poorly understood. For some infants, recovery from PN-related cholestasis may take months following cessation of PN and others may proceed to liver failure requiring transplantation.[60]

Enteral Nutrition

Trophic feeds

Because of the immaturity of the intestinal tract of premature infants, enteral feeds are not initiated in full volume and caloric density. Instead, trophic feeds, or minimal enteral feeds, are instituted optimally within the first 1 to 4 days of life. Trophic feeds are not meant to be nutritive but to instigate maturation of the intestinal wall and to encourage absorption of nutrients. The volume of the feeding is 10 to 20 mL/kg/d

Table 1
Current recommendations for established PN for premature infants less than 1000 g and 1000 to 1500 g

Nutrient/Element	<1000 g	1000–1500 g
Fluid (mL/kg/d)	140–180	120–160
Energy (kcal/kg/d)	105–115	90–100
Protein (g/kg/d)	3.5–4.0	3.2–3.8
Carbohydrate (g/100kcal)	7–14	7–14
Fat (g/kg/d)	3–4	3–4
Sodium (mg/100kcal)	38–58	38–58
Potassium (mg/100kcal)	65–100	65–100
Chloride (mg/100kcal)	59–89	59–89
Calcium (mg/kg/d)	40–80	60–80
Iron (μg/kg/d; added once per week)	100–200	100–200
Vitamin A (μg/kg/day)	280	280
Vitamin D (μg/kg/day)	4	4
Vitamin E (mg/kg/day)	2.8–3.5	2.8–3.5
Vitamin K_1 (μg/100kcal)	4–15	4–15
Ascorbate (μg/100kcal)	15–25	15–25
Thiamine (mg/kg/day)	0.48	0.48
Riboflavin (mg/kg/day)	0.56	0.56
Pyridoxine (mg/kg/day)	0.4	0.4
Niacin (mg/kg/d)	4–6.8	4–6.8
Pantothenate (mg/kg/d)	1–2	1–2
Biotin (μg/kg/d)	5–8	5–8
Folate (μg/kg/d)	56	56
Vitamin B_{12} (μg/kg/d)	0.3–0.4	0.3–0.4
Zinc (μg/kg/d)	400	250–400
Copper (μg/kg/d)	20	20
Selenium (μg/kg/d)	2	2
Manganese (μg/kg/d)	1	1
Molybdenum (μg/kg/d)	0.25	0.25
Iodine (μg/kg/d)	1	1
Chromium (μg/kg/d)	0.2	0.2

Data from Refs.[11,54,58,72]

divided into volumes given every 4 to 6 hours via gavage tube. Breast milk is preferred; either the infant's mother's expressed milk or pasteurized donor milk. If neither is available, one of the commercial premature infant formula preparations is used.[11,54,61–68]

Depending on the gestational age and birth weight of the premature infant, trophic feeds are continued for 3 to 5 days; the more immature the infant, the longer the trophic feeds are continued before initiating gradual increase in feeds to the full volume and caloric density currently recommended for optimal enteral nutrition.[11,65,67,69,70] Nutrient recommendations for established enteral feeds are summarized in Table 2.

Table 2
Current recommendations for established enteral nutrition for premature infants less than 1000 g and 1000 to 1500 g

Nutrient/Element	<1000 g	1000–1500 g
Fluid (mL/kg/d)	140–180	135–190
Energy (kcal/kg/d)	130–150	110–130
Protein (g/kg/d)	3.8–4.4	3.4–4.2
Carbohydrate (g/kg/d)	9–20	7–17
Fat (g/kg/d)	6.2–8.4	5.3–7.2
Sodium (mg/100kcal)	38–58	38–58
Potassium (mg/100kcal)	65–100	65–100
Chloride (mg/100kcal)	59–89	59–89
Calcium (mg/100kcal)	100–192	100–192
Iron (mg/kg/d)	2–4	2–4
Vitamin A (IU/100kcal)	700–1500	700–1500
Vitamin D (IU/100kcal)	150–400	150–400
Vitamin E (IU/100kcal)	6–12	6–12
Vitamin K_1 (μg/100kcal)	8–10	8–10
Ascorbate (mg/100kcal)	18–24	18–24
Thiamine (μg/100kcal)	180–240	180–240
Riboflavin (μg/100kcal)	250–360	250–360
Pyridoxine (μg/100kcal)	150–210	150–210
Niacin (mg/100kcal)	3.6–4.8	3.6–4.8
Pantothenate (mg/100kcal)	1.2–1.7	1.2–1.7
Biotin (μg/100kcal)	3.6–6	3.6–6
Folate (μg/100kcal)	25–50	25–50
Vitamin B_{12} (μg/100kcal)	0.3	0.3
Zinc (μg/100kcal)	800–1100	800–1100
Copper (μg/100kcal)	100–125	100–125
Selenium (μg/100kcal)	1.3–2.5	1.3–2.5
Manganese (μg/100kcal)	0.7–7.75	0.7–7.75
Molybdenum (μg/100kcal)	0.3	0.3
Iodine (μg/100kcal)	10–60	10–60
Chromium (μg/100kcal)	0.1–0.4	0.1–0.4
Taurine (mg/100kcal)	4.5–9.0	4.5–9.0
Carnitine (mg/100kcal)	~2.9	~2.9
Inositol (mg/100kcal)	27–67	27–67
Choline (mg/100kcal)	12–23	12–23

Data from Refs.[11,54,72]

The trophic feeds followed by the gradual increase of feeding volume and caloric density are meant to reduce the risk of developing NEC and to improve the tolerance to eventual full-volume and full-caloric-density feedings, although there is little evidence to support this practice.[11,65,67,69–71] Despite the lack of research evidence in support of such practice, clinical application of such protocols occurs in most NICUs, especially for ELBW and SGA infants.[71] **Tables 3** and **4** are examples of feeding protocols for premature infants less than 1250 g birth weight (see **Table 3**) and 1250 to 1500 g birth weight (see **Table 4**).[67,69]

Enteric feeds after NEC

Following a feeding protocol similar to that shown in **Table 3** for infants recovering from medical NEC (NEC managed without surgical intervention) is also recommended, with a paucity of research to support this recommendation. Enteral feeds for infants with surgical NEC and with SBS are generally based on feeding protocols for ELBW infants, individual infant response to enteral feeds, and surgeon preferences.

Human Breast Milk

Human breast milk is the best enteral feed for all infants, especially premature infants, with few exceptions. Mother's expressed breast milk has improved digestibility, unique immunologic components, and balanced nutritional components that specifically support growth and development.[11,30,61,64,65,68,72–75] There is strong evidence that mother's own milk may reduce the risk of NEC for premature infants.[38,69] Use of maternal expressed breast milk is associated with improved neurodevelopmental outcomes, lower incidences of late-onset sepsis and retinopathy of prematurity, and decreased incidence of adult-onset chronic diseases such as hypertension and diabetes.[61,68,73]

Donor Breast Milk

The use of donor milk, from established human breast milk banks, is increasingly seen in NICUs when mother's milk is not available as an alternative to commercial

Table 3
A feeding protocol for premature infants less than 1250 g. Use unfortified mother's expressed breast milk, donor milk, or premature infant formula (20 cal/oz)

Day	Total Volume (mL/kg/d)	Interval, Volume Divided Equally (h)
Day 1	10	Every 6
Days 2–3	10	Every 4
Day 4	10	Every 3
Days 5–7	20	Every 3
Day 8	40	Every 3
Day 9	60	Every 3
Day 10	80	Every 3
Day 11	100	Every 3
Day 12	100 Fortify to 22 cal/oz	Every 3
Day 13	120	Every 3
Day 14	120 Fortify to 24 cal/oz	Every 3
Day 15	140 Discontinue PN and PICC	Every 3
Day 16	150–160	Every 3

Abbreviation: PICC, peripherally inserted central catheter.
  Data from Refs.[65,67,69]

Table 4
A feeding protocol for premature infants 1250 to 1500 g. Use unfortified mother's expressed breast milk, donor milk, or premature infant formula (20 cal/oz)

Day	Total Volume (mL/kg/d)	Interval, Volume Divided Equally (h)
Day 1–3	10–20	Every 3
Days 4–5	30–40	Every 3
Day 6	50–60	Every 3
Days 7	70–80	Every 3
Day 8	90–100	Every 3
Day 9	100–110	Every 3
Day 10	100–110 Fortify to 22 cal/oz	Every 3
Day 11	110–120	Every 3
Day 12	120–130 Fortify to 24 cal/oz	Every 3
Day 13	130–140 Discontinue PN and PICC	Every 3
Day 14	140–150	Every 3
Day 15	150–160	Every 3

Data from Refs.[65,67,69]

premature formula products. Both the World Health Organization and the American Academy of Pediatrics endorse donor milk use when mother's milk is not available.[76]

Donor milk is collected from mothers who are either breast feeding concurrently or have recently weaned infants and have been rigorously screened for infectious diseases. Donor milk is lower in protein than term breast milk and has lost many of the bioactive components that provide immunoprotection. There is no evidence that donor milk provides protection from NEC or late-onset sepsis or that it provides any of the associated benefits from expressed mother's milk. There is an association between lower incidences of NEC for infants fed donor milk compared with formula; however, donor milk is associated with a slower rate of growth.[77] Further research is needed to discover better pasteurization methods to prevent transmission of disease but preserve the bioactive components of donor milk.[61,62,64,68,69,74,78,79]

Breast Milk Fortifiers and Premature Infant Formulas

Premature infants need more protein, fat, energy, electrolytes, minerals, and micronutrients than are provided in unfortified breast milk (see **Table 2**). Breast milk obtained in the first few weeks following preterm delivery has more of these basic nutrients than breast milk following term delivery, but not in sufficient quantities to support the additional requirements of premature infants for adequate growth and development.[11,30,70,80–88] Increasing protein in enteral feeds is of special importance, because of rapid brain and somatic growth. Breast milk fortifiers, both in powder and liquid form and derived from either cow or human milk, improve protein, energy, and micronutrient intake and are associated with tolerance and enhanced growth. Powdered formula (premature, transitional, or term powdered formula) is also added to increase protein and caloric content in breast milk to recommended levels for gestational age/weight.[53,68,69,82,83,89] If no breast milk is available, there are several commercially prepared premature infant formulas available that are formulated to closely follow currently recommended nutrient content, as summarized in **Table 2**. Soy-based formulas are not recommended for premature infants because of increased incidence of osteopenia of prematurity.[90]

Assessment of Growth in Response to Nutritional Support

Weight, head circumference, and length

Body weight is the most commonly performed (usually daily), and the most readily accepted as accurate, determinant of growth in NICUs.[22,91,92] Digital bed and portable scales are accurate to the nearest gram.

Head circumference is determined by applying a paper or plasticized paper measurement tape firmly around the head above the supraorbital ridges, over the most prominent part of the frontal bulge and around the part of the occiput that gives the maximum circumference.[12] Head circumference measurements are done weekly to track brain growth response in normally developing premature infants.

Length measurement is most typically crown to heel (crown-heel) measurement. The most accurate length measurement is performed weekly with a length board specific for premature infants, such as the Premie Length Board (O'Leary, Ellard Instrumentation Ltd, Seattle, WA).[12,93]

Growth charts

Growth charts that include growth curves for weight, head circumference, and length have been developed using compiled data from estimated fetal weight for gestation and birth weights of early fetuses and premature infants at each gestation. Two growth charts in current use by NICUs in the United States are the Fenton premature growth chart[94] and the Olsen growth chart.[95]

Body composition measurements

Recent research is showing increasing evidence that weight and length should be used jointly to provide more accurate assessment of premature growth. Evidence suggests that the body composition of premature infants tends more toward increased adipose deposits than lean body mass and brain growth. More evidence is showing that weight-for-length or a ponderal index (g/cm^3) should become standard measurements in NICUs so as to monitor body composition rather than just weight gain.[22,83,92,96,97]

Effect of Nutrition During Initial Hospitalization of Premature Infants on Later Adulthood

Evidence is mounting that premature infants are predisposed to obesity in later childhood and/or adulthood as an effect of early and rapid weight gain, often referred to as catch-up growth. There is concern that rapid catch-up growth for premature infants with growth restriction is increasingly associated with obesity, diabetes, hypertension, proteinuria, and hyperuricemia (abnormally high blood uric acid level) in later life.[10,43,98] Nutritional support for infants in the NICU not only needs to meet the needs for growth but also support reduction of later adult-onset chronic disease. Providing consistent nutritional support from birth throughout hospitalization is the ideal way to attain and promote this goal.[71,96]

SUMMARY

Providing optimal nutritional support for premature infants in the NICU is an important challenge that neonatal health care providers face on a daily basis. Of primary importance is the challenge of providing optimal nutrition in a safe and efficacious manner to infants who need to continue to grow and develop at a time when their anatomy and physiologic functioning are not mature enough to cope with the nutrients provided. In addition, nutrition must support not only weight gain but also brain growth and lean body mass so as to minimize neurodevelopmental deficits and decrease risks of developing chronic diseases during later childhood into adulthood. Ongoing research is needed to continue to support the technology, nutritional products and supplements, and the evidence-based practices that have already been developed to provide optimal nutritional support for the smallest patients.

REFERENCES

1. Botet F, Figueras-Aloy J, Miracle-Echegoyen X, et al. Trends in survival among extremely-low-birthweight infants (less than 1000 g) without significant bronchopulmonary dysplasia. BMC Pediatr 2012;12(63):1–7.
2. Dani C, Poggi C. Nutrition and bronchopulmonary dysplasia. J Matern Fetal Neonatal Med 2012;25(S3):37–40.
3. Ehrenkranz RA, Das A, Wrage LA, et al. Early nutrition mediates the influence of severity of illness on extremely LBW infants. Pediatr Res 2011;69(6):522–9.
4. Franz AR, Pohlandt F, Bode H, et al. Intrauterine, early neonatal, and postdischarge growth and neurodevelopmental outcome at 5.4 years in extremely preterm infants after intensive neonatal nutritional support. Pediatrics 2009;123(1): e101–9.
5. Geary CA, Caskey MA, Malloy MH. Improved growth and decreased morbidities in <1000 g neonates after early management changes. J Perinatol 2008;28: 347–53.
6. Hintz SR, Bann CM, Ambalavanan N, et al. Predicting time to hospital discharge for extremely preterm infants. Pediatrics 2010;125:e148–54.
7. Kobaly K, Schluchter M, Minich N, et al. Outcomes of extremely low birth weight (<1 kg) and extremely low gestational age (<28 weeks) infants with bronchopulmonary dysplasia: effects of practice changes in 2000-2003. Pediatrics 2008; 121:73–81.
8. Kugelman A, Bader D, Lerner-Geva L, et al. Poor outcomes at discharge among extremely premature infants. Arch Pediatr Adolesc Med 2012;891:E1–8.
9. Limperopoulos C, Soul JS, Gauvreau K, et al. Late gestation cerebellar growth is rapid and impeded by premature birth. Pediatrics 2005;115:688–93.
10. Barker DJ. The origins of the developmental origins theory. J Intern Med 2007; 261(5):412–7.
11. Ziegler EE. Meeting the nutritional needs of the low-birth-weight infant. Ann Nutr Metab 2011;58(Suppl 1):8–18.
12. Ehrenkranz RA, Dusick AM, Vohr B, et al. Growth in the neonatal intensive care unit influences neurodevelopmental and growth outcomes of extremely low birth weight infants. Pediatrics 2006;117:1253–61.
13. Embleton NE, Pang N, Cooke RJ. Postnatal malnutrition and growth retardation: an inevitable consequence of current recommendations in preterm infants? Pediatrics 2001;107(2):270–4.
14. Fanaroff AA, Stoll BJ, Wright LL, et al. Trends in neonatal morbidity and mortality for very low birthweight infants. Am J Obstet Gynecol 2007;196(2):147.e1–8.

15. Henriksen C, Khan S, Weishuhn K, et al. Growth and nutrient intake among very-low-birth-weight infants fed fortified human milk during hospitalisation. Br J Nutr 2009;102:1179–86.
16. Limperopoulos C. Extreme prematurity, cerebellar injury, and autism. Semin Pediatr Neurol 2010;17:25–9.
17. Longo S, Bollani L, Decembrino L, et al. Short-term and long-term sequelae in intrauterine growth retardation (IUGR). J Matern Fetal Neonatal Med 2013; 26(3):222–5.
18. Cooke R. Postnatal growth in preterm infants: have we got it right? J Perinatol 2005;25:S12–4.
19. Roggero P, Gianni ML, Amato O, et al. Postnatal growth failure in preterm infants: recovery of growth and body composition after term. Early Hum Dev 2008;84:555–9.
20. Stoll BJ, Hansen NI, Bell EF, et al. Neonatal outcomes of extremely preterm infants from the NICHD Neonatal Research Network. Pediatrics 2010;126(3): 443–56.
21. Tan M, Abernethy L, Cooke R. Improving head growth in preterm infants a randomised controlled trial II: MRI and developmental outcomes in the first year. Arch Dis Child Fetal Neonatal Ed 2007;93:F342–6.
22. Bhatia J. Growth curves: how to best measure growth of the preterm infant. J Pediatr 2013;162(Suppl 3):S2–6.
23. Blackburn ST. Maternal, fetal, and neonatal physiology: a clinical perspective. 4th edition. St Louis (MO): Saunders/Elsevier; 2013.
24. Berseth CL. Development and physiology of the gastrointestinal tract. In: Thureen P, Hay W, editors. Neonatal nutrition and metabolism. 2nd edition. New York: Cambridge University Press; 2006. p. 1071–85.
25. Dimmitt RA, Sibley E. Developmental anatomy and physiology of the gastrointestinal tract. In: Gleason CA, Devaskar SU, editors. Avery's diseases of the newborn. 9th edition. Philadelphia: Saunders/Elsevier; 2012. p. 973–8.
26. Berseth CL. The intestine as a neuro-endocrine organ. In: Polin RA, editor. Gastroenterology and nutrition: neonatology questions and controversies. Philadelphia: Saunders/Elsevier; 2008. p. 111–20.
27. Moore KL, Persaud T, Torchia MG. The developing human: clinically oriented embryology. 9th edition. Philadelphia: Saunders/Elsevier; 2013.
28. Arboleya S, Binetti A, Salazar N, et al. Establishment and development of intestinal microbiota in preterm neonates. FEMS Microbiol Ecol 2012;79(3):763–72.
29. Jacobi SK, Odle J. Nutritional factors influencing intestinal health of the neonate. Adv Nutr 2012;3(5):687–96.
30. Kashyap S. Enteral intake for very low birth weight infants: what should the composition be? Semin Perinatol 2007;31:74–82.
31. Neu J. Gastrointestinal development and meeting the nutritional needs of premature infants. Am J Clin Nutr 2007;85(2):629S–34S.
32. Neville MC, McManaman JL. Milk secretion and composition. In: Thureen PJ, Hay WW, editors. Neonatal nutrition and metabolism. 2nd edition. Philadelphia: Cambridge University Press; 2006. p. 377–89.
33. Field DG, Hillemeier AC. Fetal and neonatal intestinal motility. In: Polin RA, Fox WW, Abman SH, editors. Fetal and neonatal physiology, vol. 2, 4th edition. Philadelphia: Saunders/Elsevier; 2011. p. 1226–9.
34. Omari TI, Rudolph CD. Gastrointestinal motility. In: Polin RA, Fox WW, Abman SH, editors. Fetal and neonatal physiology, vol. 2, 4th edition. Philadelphia: Saunders/Elsevier; 2011. p. 1212–25.

35. Gutierrez IM, Kang KH, Jaksic T. Neonatal short bowel syndrome. Semin Fetal Neonatal Med 2011;16(3):157–63.

36. Lucchini R, Bizzarri B, Giampietro S, et al. Feeding intolerance in preterm infants. How to understand the warning signs. J Matern Fetal Neonatal Med 2011;24(S1):72–4.

37. Emami CN, Petrosyan M, Giuliani S, et al. Role of the host defense system and intestinal microbial flora in the pathogenesis of necrotizing enterocolitis. Surg Infect (Larchmt) 2009;10(5):407–17.

38. Neu J, Douglas-Escobar M. Necrotizing enterocolitis: pathogenesis, clinical care and prevention. In: Neu J, Polin RA, editors. Gastroenterology and nutrition: neonatology questions and controversies. Philadelphia: Saunders/Elsevier; 2008. p. 281–91.

39. Kuppala VS, Meinzen-Derr J, Morrow AL, et al. Prolonged initial empirical antibiotic treatment is associated with adverse outcomes in premature infants. J Pediatr 2011;159(5):720–5.

40. Tzialla C, Borghesi A, Perotti GF, et al. Use and misuse of antibiotics in the neonatal intensive care unit. J Matern Fetal Neonatal Med 2012;25(S4):27–9.

41. Cotten CM, Taylor S, Stoll B, et al. Prolonged duration of initial empirical antibiotic treatment is associated with increased rates of necrotizing enterocolitis and death for extremely low birth weight infants. Pediatrics 2009;123(1):58–66.

42. Chen MK. Short bowel syndrome and intestinal tissue engineering. In: Neu J, Polin RA, editors. Gastroenterology and nutrition: neonatology questions and controversies. Philadelphia: Saunders/Elsevier; 2008. p. 310–7.

43. Abitobol CL, Rodriguez MM. The long-term renal and cardiovascular consequences of prematurity. Nat Rev Nephrol 2012;8:265–74.

44. Sweeney WE Jr, Avner ED. Embryogenesis and anatomic development of the kidney. In: Polin RA, Fox WW, Abman SH, editors. Fetal and neonatal physiology, vol. 2, 4th edition. Philadelphia: Saunders; 2011. p. 1307–16.

45. Bueva A, Guignard JP. Renal function in preterm infants. Pediatr Res 1994; 36(5):572–7.

46. Gallini F, Maggio L, Romagnoli C, et al. Progression of renal function in preterm neonates with gestational age ≤32 weeks. Pediatr Nephrol 2000;15:119–24.

47. Janjua HS, Batisky DL. Renal vascular disease in the newborn. In: Taeush HW, Ballard RA, Gleason CA, editors. Avery's diseases of the newborn. 9th edition. Philadelphia: Elsevier Saunders; 2011. p. 1235–44.

48. Aly H, Davies J, El-Dib M, et al. Renal function is impaired in small for gestational age premature infants. J Matern Fetal Neonatal Med 2013;26(4):388–91.

49. Chevalier RL, Norwood VF. Functional development of the kidney in utero. In: Polin RA, Fox WW, Abman SH, editors. Fetal and neonatal physiology, vol. 2, 4th edition. Philadelphia: Saunders; 2011. p. 1317–24.

50. Cuzzolin L, Fanos V, Pinna B, et al. Postnatal renal function in preterm newborns: a role of diseases, drugs and therapeutic interventions. Pediatr Nephrol 2006; 21:931–8.

51. Biasini A, Marvulli L, Neri E, et al. Growth and neurological outcome in ELBW preterms fed with human milk and extra-protein supplementation as routine practice: do we need further evidence? J Matern Fetal Neonatal Med 2012; 25(S4):64–6.

52. Cleper R. Mechanisms of compensatory renal growth. Pediatr Endocrinol Rev 2012;10(1):152–63.

53. Arslanoglu S, Moro GE, Ziegler EE. Adjustable fortification of human milk fed to preterm infants: does it make a difference? J Perinatol 2006;26(10):614–21.

54. Tudehope D, Fewtrell M, Kashyap S, et al. Nutritional needs of the micropreterm infant. J Pediatr 2013;162(Suppl 3):S72–80.
55. Arslanoglu S, Moro GE, Ziegler EE. Preterm infants fed fortified human milk receive less protein than they need. J Perinatol 2009;29:489–92.
56. Hans BM, Pylipow M, Long JD, et al. Nutritional practices in the neonatal intensive care unit: analysis of a 2006 neonatal nutrition survey. Pediatrics 2009;123:51–7.
57. Ogilvy-Stuart AL, Beardsall K. Management of hyperglycaemia in the preterm infant. Arch Dis Child Fetal Neonatal Ed 2010;95:F126–31.
58. Heird WC. Intravenous feeding. In: Thureen PJ, Hay WW, editors. Neonatal nutrition and metabolism. 2nd edition. New York: Cambridge University Press; 2008. p. 312–31.
59. Armentrout D. Glucose management. In: Verklan MT, Walden M, editors. Core curriculum for neonatal intensive care nursing. St Louis (MO): Saunders/Elsevier; 2010. p. 172–81.
60. Davis MK, Andres JM. Cholestasis in neonates and infants. In: Neu J, Polin RA, editors. Gastroenterology and nutrition: neonatology questions and controversies. Philadelphia: Saunders/Elsevier; 2008. p. 135–63.
61. American Academy of Pediatrics, Section on Breastfeeding. Breastfeeding and the use of human milk. Pediatrics 2012;129(3):e827–41.
62. Arslanoglu S, Ziegler EE, Moro GE, et al. Donor human milk in preterm infant feeding: evidence and recommendations. J Perinat Med 2010;38(4):347–51.
63. Bertino E, Giuliani F, Occhi L, et al. Benefits of donor human milk for preterm infants: current evidence. Early Hum Dev 2009;85(Suppl 10):S9–10.
64. Hamosh M. Human milk composition and function in the infant. In: Polin RA, Fox WW, Abman SH, editors. Fetal and neonatal physiology, vol. 1, 4th edition. Philadelphia: Saunders/Elsevier; 2011. p. 323–33.
65. Morgan J, Bombell S, McGuire W. Early trophic feeding versus enteral fasting for very preterm or very low birth weight infants. Cochrane Database Syst Rev 2013;(3):CD000504.
66. Neu J. Gastrointestinal maturation and implications for infant feeding. Early Hum Dev 2007;83:767–75.
67. Morgan J, Young L, McGuire W. Slow advancement of enteral feed volumes to prevent necrotising enterocolitis in very low birth weight infants. Cochrane Database Syst Rev 2013;(3):CD001241.
68. Underwood MA. Human milk for the premature infant. Pediatr Clin North Am 2013;60(1):189–207.
69. Groh-Wargo S, Sapsford A. Enteral nutrition support of the preterm infant in the neonatal intensive care unit. Nutr Clin Pract 2009;24(3):363–76.
70. Parish A, Bhatia J. Feeding strategies in the ELBW infant. J Perinatol 2008;28: S18–20.
71. Corrpeleijn WE, Vermeulen MJ, van den Akker CH, et al. Feeding very-low-birth-weight infants: our aspirations versus the reality in practice. Ann Nutr Metab 2011;58(Suppl 1):20–9.
72. Kleinman RE, Committee on Nutrition, editors. Pediatric nutrition handbook. Elk Grove Village (IL): American Academy of Pediatrics; 2009.
73. Schanler RJ. Outcomes of human milk-fed premature infants. Semin Perinatol 2011;35:29–33.
74. Tudehope DI. Human milk and the nutritional needs of preterm infants. J Pediatr 2013;162(Suppl 3):S17–25.
75. Yeung MY. Influence of early postnatal nutritional management on oxidative stress and antioxidant defence in extreme prematurity. Acta Paediatr 2006;95(2):153–63.

76. Parker MG, Barrero-Castillero A, Corwin BK, et al. Pasteurized human donor milk use among US level 3 neonatal intensive care units. J Hum Lact 2013;29(3):381–9.
77. Bhatia J. Human milk and premature infant. Ann Nutr Metab 2013;62(Suppl 3): 8–14.
78. Schanler RJ. Human milk supplementation for preterm infants. Acta Paediatr 2005;94:64–7.
79. Schanler RJ. Fortified human milk for premature infants. In: Thureen PJ, Hay WW, editors. Neonatal nutrition and metabolism. 2nd edition. New York: Cambridge University Press; 2006. p. 401–8.
80. Kashyap S, Heird WC. Protein and amino acid metabolism and requirements. In: Polin RA, Fox WW, Abman SH, editors. Fetal and neonatal physiology, vol. 1, 4th edition. Philadelphia: Saunders/Elsevier; 2011. p. 603–15.
81. Maggio L, Cota F, Lauriola V, et al. Effects of high versus standard early protein intake on growth of extremely low birth weight infants. J Pediatr Gastroenterol Nutr 2007;44:124–9.
82. Maggio L, Costa S, Gallini F. Human milk fortifiers in very low birth weight infants. Early Hum Dev 2009;85:S59–61.
83. Moya F, Sisk PM, Walsh KR, et al. A new liquid human milk fortifier and linear growth in preterm infants. Pediatrics 2012;130(4):e928–35.
84. Reis BB, Hall RT, Schanler R, et al. Enhanced growth of preterm infants fed a new powdered human milk fortifier: a randomized, controlled trial. Pediatrics 2000;106:581–8.
85. Thureen P, Heird W. Protein and energy requirements of the preterm/low birth-weight (LBW) infant. Pediatr Res 2005;57(5):95R–8R.
86. Williford A, Pare L, Carlson G. Bone mineral metabolism in the neonate: calcium, phosphorus, magnesium, and alkaline phosphatase. Neonatal Netw 2008;27(1): 57–63.
87. Zachariassen G, Faerk J, Grytter C, et al. Nutrient enrichment of mother's milk and growth of very preterm infants after hospital discharge. Pediatrics 2011; 127:e995–1003.
88. Ziegler EE, Lucas A, Moro GE. Nutrition of the very low birthweight infant, vol. 43. Philadelphia: Nestec/Lippincott Williams & Wilkins; 1999.
89. Cooke R. Adjustable fortification of human milk fed to preterm infants. J Perinatol 2006;26(10):591–2.
90. Bhatia J, Greer F, American Academy of Pediatrics Committee on Nutrition. Use of soy protein-based formulas in infant feeding. Pediatrics 2008;121(5):1062–8.
91. Belfort MB, Gillman MW, Buka SL, et al. Preterm infant linear growth and adiposity gain: trade-offs for later weight status and intelligence quotient. J Pediatr 2013;163(6):1564–9.e2. Available at: http://www.jpeds.com.
92. Olsen IE, Lawson ML, Meinzen-Derr J, et al. Use of a body proportionality index for growth assessment of preterm infants. J Pediatr 2009;154:486–91.
93. Moyer-Mileur LJ. Anthropometric and laboratory assessment of very low birth weight infants: the most helpful measurements and why. Semin Perinatol 2007;31:96–103.
94. Fenton TR, Nasser R, Eliasziw M, et al. Validating the weight gain of preterm infants between the reference growth curve of the fetus and the term infant. BMC Pediatr 2013;13:92–102.
95. Olsen IE, Groveman S, Lawson ML, et al. New intrauterine growth curves based on United States data. Pediatrics 2010;125:e214–24.
96. Lapillonne A, Griffin IJ. Feeding preterm infants today for later metabolic and cardiovascular outcomes. J Pediatr 2013;162(Suppl 3):S7–16.

97. Stokes TA, Holston A, Olsen C, et al. Preterm infants of lower gestational age at birth have greater waist circumference-length ratio and ponderal index at term age than preterm infants of higher gestational ages. J Pediatr 2012;161(4): 735–42.

98. Barker DJ. The malnourished baby and infant: relationship with type 2 diabetes. Br Med Bull 2001;60(1):69–88.

Nutrition in the Pediatric Population in the Intensive Care Unit

Judy Verger, RN, PhD, CRNP, CCRN[a,b,c,*]

KEYWORDS

- Nutrition • Critically ill child • Nutritional disorders • Child • Intensive care unit

KEY POINTS

- Critically ill infants and children have an increase in metabolic needs and lower macronutrient stores.
- For any hospitalized child, growth assessment is vitally important, and documenting baseline nutrition parameters including body weight, length/height, and body mass index provides guidance for nutritional support.
- The energy requirements for the critically ill child are highly individualized and may vary widely.
- The immunoglobulins available in human milk support a wide range of bacteriostatic and bactericidal activity.
- Although brief nutritional inadequacies may have limited consequences, if adequate oral intake is not expected within 24 to 48 hours of admission, alternative methods should be sought.
- Parenteral nutrition is used in the pediatric intensive care unit when the enteral route cannot be used or is unable to provide sufficient calories.

INTRODUCTION

Nutrition is an essential component of patient management in the pediatric intensive care unit (PICU). Critically ill infants and children have an increase in metabolic needs and lower macronutrient stores inherent in infancy and childhood. In addition, the added nutritional complexities of critical illness make providing adequate nutrition

No Disclosures.

[a] Pediatric Acute Care Nurse Practitioner Program, Critical Care Department, School of Nursing, Children's Hospital of Philadelphia, University of Pennsylvania, 17 Ridings Way, Chadds Ford, PA 19317, USA; [b] Pediatric Clinical Nurse Specialist Program, Critical Care Department, School of Nursing, Children's Hospital of Philadelphia, University of Pennsylvania, 17 Ridings Way, Chadds Ford, PA 19317, USA; [c] Neonatal Clinical Nurse Specialist Program, Critical Care Department, School of Nursing, Children's Hospital of Philadelphia, University of Pennsylvania, 17 Ridings Way, Chadds Ford, PA 19317, USA

* 17 Ridings Way, Chadds Ford, PA 19317.

E-mail address: Jtv2526@yahoo.com

particularly difficult. Undernourished states are a common consequence of disease and its treatment. Although a few recent studies challenge assumptions, the significance of nutrition support for hospitalized patients has been well documented.[1–7] Delivery of acceptable nutrient amounts is linked with enhanced clinical outcomes, including improved wound healing and tissue integrity.[7–15] Higher calorie and protein intake is associated with positive protein balance in children who are ventilated mechanically.[8,16–18] In addition, increased delivery of nutrition is linked to reduced infection rates, length of hospital stay, and mortality, especially when nutrition protocols are in place.[1,8,13,15,19]

Malnutrition has been reported at admission and during hospitalization in critically ill children since the 1980s.[20–27] Two of the first widely disseminated studies were completed by Pollack and colleagues.[25,26] These investigators noted a 20% occurrence of chronic and acute malnutrition. A recent study confirmed that rates for suboptimal nutrition remain high in PICUs worldwide.[28] This international point prevalence study included 31 intensive care units (ICUs), and found that 30% of all PICU patients demonstrate signs of malnutrition.

The trajectory of critical illness varies and is a multifactorial, heterogeneous disease process. Hypermetabolism leads to a shortfall in energy, and simultaneous changes in micronutrient and macronutrient needs. Body storage sites, especially muscles, are depleted for energy to support the immune system and other key body functions. Despite this catabolism, the contraction of muscle fibers associated with mechanical work is an energy-demanding process. With muscle wasting, respiratory insufficiency may lead to delayed weaning from mechanical ventilation.[29] Gastrointestinal (GI) dysfunction is commonly reported in critically ill patients.[30,31] The motility of the GI tract diminishes almost immediately, triggered by sympathetic stimulation and the inflammatory response connected to injury.[32] Alterations in the GI tract place the patient at risk for systemic infections by translocation of the GI flora into the systemic circulation. Acute lower respiratory infections have been associated with undernutrition and zinc deficiency.[33] Malnourished patients often have prolonged hospitalizations and increased hospital costs.[22,24,34,35]

Poor nutrition status accompanies many chronic childhood diseases. Conditions such as congenital heart disease (CHD), oncologic disorders, significant neurologic dysfunction, and other common chronic conditions contribute to the risk of undernutrition. Infants with CHD have demonstrated the presence of growth failure in all age groups and in all stages of repair.[20,36] Patients with CHD have a 3.6 times higher chance of not reaching satisfactory caloric intake when matched against subjects without CHD.[20] Factors leading to energy deficiency in children with cancer include insufficient intake, increased metabolic rate, altered physical activity, and inflammation.[37] Those children with conditions that include severe motor disability are at higher risk of undernutrition.[38] In addition, infants with brainstem injury often have feeding difficulties.[39]

An imbalance of energy and nutrient equation leads to nutrition related consequences. Children with injury or sepsis or those who are admitted to the ICU in a malnourished state are particularly at risk and require the highest priority. Although the metabolic response in critical illness is unavoidable, provision of adequate calories and protein based on patient size and metabolic needs is crucial.[40]

DETERMINING NUTRITIONAL NEEDS

A thorough assessment of the critically ill child is required to inform the plan for nutritional support. The American Society of Parenteral and Enteral Nutrition (ASPEN) nutritional support guidelines for critically ill children recommend that children undergo nutrition screening to identify those with existing malnutrition and those nutritionally at risk.[13] The Joint Commission requires assessment of nutritional risk within 24 hours of hospital admission.[41] Those not at risk on admission should be regularly rescreened, as significant protein and energy depletion in patients hospitalized for longer than 7 to 10 days has been demonstrated.[42] Added risk is also related to the longer duration the patient has been without adequate nutrition. When screening measures identify risk of malnutrition, a formal assessment is warranted.

No sole assessment measure is adequate to provide a complete picture of the nutritional status of sick infants and children. A systematic appraisal of the child's physical examination findings, a review of relevant diagnostics, and an awareness of the metabolic consequences of the child disease are essential. Clinical and biochemical assessment strategies provide specific information to support nutritional prescription. In addition, an evaluation of energy expenditure can be an important asset in guiding the nutrition plan.

The first step in nutritional risk assessment is a careful history. Accurate and clinically relevant nutritional assessment provides important guidance.[32] Historical growth data, hospitalizations, surgical procedures, and acute and chronic conditions, especially those that have GI sequelae and feeding difficulties, are important to note. Because of their effect on intake, identifying prior sensory and fine motor dysfunction and chewing and swallowing difficulties is important. In addition, any recent weight loss or decreases in nutrient intake are key indicators of nutrition risk.

The physical examination is useful in establishing nutrition status. Some of the first visual signs of protein malnutrition are seen in rapidly growing tissues.[42,43] Skin is thin, dull, and dry in appearance. Hair is brittle and falls out easily. The abdomen may appear large because of the lack of strength in the overlying muscles. For a child with severe malnutrition, legs may be edematous. The overall appearance of the child is one of muscle wasting.

For any hospitalized child, growth assessment is vitally important. Documenting baseline nutrition parameters provides guidance for nutrition support. Body weight, length/height, and body mass index are staples of a nutrition assessment strategy. Weight loss is the best single physical examination predictor of malnutrition risk. When measuring weight, use of the same scale with sequential measurements is important. When interpreting weight, fluid retention and diuresis may mask nutrition-related weight changes.[44–46] Length is measured in children younger than 2 years. Height, using a stadiometer, is required for children older than 3 years. Height estimation is also possible through measurement of knee height.[32] Nutrition-related reductions in linear growth are often attributed to chronic malnutrition. Body mass index uses weight and length in children older than 2 years as a screening tool for body fat.[47] Relevant growth chart based on age and sex are used to evaluate measurements against a standard and plot growth trajectory. In 2006 the US Centers for Disease Control and Prevention (CDC) recommended the use of the World Health Organization (WHO) growth charts for children younger than 24 months.[48] CDC growth charts are still recommended for children from 2 to 19 years of age. Children aged 24 to 35 months can be charted on either growth chart, depending on whether there is a need to compare growth measurements against past growth or future growth.

With children at risk, additional anthropometrics are warranted. In many institutions, registered dieticians measure and compute arm circumference, arm muscle area, arm muscle circumference, and triceps skin-fold thickness. These measurements can provide additional information related to body composition, including fat and protein stores. A reduction in midarm circumference is linked to negative nitrogen balance.[49]

Biochemical markers such as albumin and prealbumin are commonly used to reflect visceral serum protein. Albumin has a half-life of 14 to 20 days. Given its long half-life, albumin's clinical limitations make it an imperfect marker for evaluating the nutrition status of the critically ill child. Prealbumin is a stable circulating glycoprotein synthesized in the liver, and has been used successfully as an indicator of protein status.[44,50] Prealbumin has a half-life of approximately 24 to 48 hours and correlates with nitrogen balance. Despite some clinical limitations, prealbumin is thought to be helpful in informing the adequacy of protein replacement. Critical illness in itself has a specific association to plasma proteins. C-reactive protein (CRP) has a negative relationship, which can be used to help differentiate a nutrition-related cause of prealbumin response.

Measurement of energy expenditure has the ability to influence nutritional prescription. Analysis of inspiratory and expiratory gas concentrations to determine oxygen consumption and carbon dioxide (CO_2) production provides an evaluation of intracellular metabolism. According to the ASPEN clinical guidelines, "energy expenditure should be assessed throughout the course of illness to determine energy needs of critically ill children."[13(p263)] These guidelines support the use of indirect calorimetry, given that standard formulas are erratic in their ability to match measured energy expenditure. In many institutions, indirect calorimetry is used at the bedside to quantify energy expenditure and drive estimates of caloric needs.[51] Unfortunately, accessibility of necessary equipment and staff with appropriate expertise in the use of indirect calorimetry is unavailable in many PICUs.

Energy Needs

The energy requirements of a critically ill child are highly individualized and may vary widely. Because the child's metabolism dictates energy needs, whatever changes metabolic response affects the child's need for and use of nutrients. The extent to which energy requirements are met depends on energy intake and absorption.

Metabolic variations exist throughout infancy and childhood. Brain metabolism drives the largest percentage of energy expenditure and, therefore, energy needs.[42] The infant's brain size is proportionally larger than that of older children, and contributes 60% of energy needs compared with 25% in adults. In addition, unlike adults, infants and children have caloric needs for growth.

Determining the caloric needs of infants and children often starts with estimating resting energy expenditure (REE). Indirect calorimetry provides the most accurate measurement of energy expenditure. Many institutions, however, routinely estimate caloric needs by computing REE. Although these formulas diverge from measured energy expenditure, they provide an initial estimate of caloric needs. The Dietary Reference Standards offer energy requirements by age.[42] These estimates provide dietary guidelines for caloric intake to maintain energy balance. Other equations such as the WHO and the Schofield equation also provide estimates of caloric needs.[52]

For sick infants and children, "factors" are often used to quantify the impact that stress and activity (or inactivity) have on a child's energy needs. REE can be multiplied by a factor of 1.5 to 1.6 for a moderately stressed critically ill child with sepsis or acute respiratory failure. A factor of 1.0 or 1.2 is generally sufficient for a ventilated patient with no growth failure. Stress factors higher than 2 are typically reserved for children with burns. Consideration should also be given to children with decreased metabolic demands such as those who are sedated or chemically paralyzed, or whose respiratory effort is supported fully by mechanical ventilation.

Despite the common use of formulas, concordance with energy expenditure has not been shown.[53–58] These results are a reminder to the clinician that caution is needed when using formulas to determine energy needs. To prevent inappropriate caloric intake, reassessment of the child's nutrition status is imperative.

Although undernutrition is of significant concern in the PICU excessive calories are also worrisome in light of the potential physiologic consequences.[59,60] Overfeeding occurs when the amount of calories exceeds the calories needed for metabolic homeostasis. Unnecessary calories have the potential to increase CO_2 production. High carbohydrate intake increases the respiratory quotient and may negatively affect the critically ill child's ventilatory status.

Macronutrient Needs

Protein, fat, and carbohydrates are the macronutrients that provide the energy to perform all body functions. The amount, source, and density of these macronutrients affect nutritional status. Guidelines for the dosing of nutrients have been offered by several organizations. In the United States, the Food and Nutrition Board, National Institutes of Medicine of the National Academies provides current standards.[61] Recommendations are framed within the context of dietary recommended intakes (DRI). These reference values are divided into 3 levels. Recommended daily allowances (RDA), last revised in the 1990s, are dietary amounts that meet the needs of more than 97% of the population for age and sex. Adequate intakes (AI) are based a review of limited data, and reflect values that meet the average child's needs based on age and sex. Upper limit intake (URI) identifies the maximum amount recommended for a particular nutrient.

Protein supplies 4 calories per gram to the diet. Protein and its derivatives contribute structurally to hormones, cell membranes, blood transport molecules, and collagen. Proteins consist of complex amino acid configurations joined by peptide bonds. Provision of adequate protein supports continuous protein turnover (degradation and resynthesis). With protein turnover, amino acids are available for redistribution away from skeletal muscle to acute-phase reactants such as CRP and fibrinogen.[62] The guidelines for protein administration are based on AI recommendations for infants and RDA for children aged 1 to 18 years. The AI intake for infants is based on an evaluation of human milk.

For sick children, increasing amounts of protein may be needed. Protein catabolism appears to peak at 8 to 14 days after injury. Patients with intractable diarrhea, chest tubes with substantial drainage, and large blood loss are especially in need of added dietary protein. In patients with severe burns, higher dietary protein intake increases outcomes.[63] Oversupply of protein can also be toxic and may be detected by an increase in blood urea nitrogen, an increase in osmolarity, and acidosis.

Nonprotein calories are delivered in the form of carbohydrates and fat. Carbohydrates contribute 4 calories per gram and provide the major source of energy for fuel. Carbohydrates are especially important to the brain and the nervous system. In the well nourished, carbohydrates prevent protein from being used for energy. Carbohydrates supply nearly half the total caloric intake. AI amounts are recommended for infants. Although carbohydrates are an essential component of the diet, early aggressive high glucose concentrations may be detrimental to patients under critical care.[64,65]

Fat provides 9 calories per gram for energy to support body function. Fat is essential for cell adhesiveness and, therefore, skin integrity and wound healing. Fat also contributes to the immune system and brain growth. Lipids can be administered to the child as long-chain triglycerides (LCT), such as soybean and safflower oils, or as medium-chain triglycerides (MCT) such as fish oil. MCT oil is appealing because it is less complex to digest, making it more readily available for energy.

Fat supports the body's need for essential fatty acids. A minimum level of 0.3% to 0.56% calories from linoleic as linolenic is necessary to avoid fatty acid deficiency. Growth can be maintained with more than 21% of diet from fat.[42] The AI recommendation for total fat in infants aged 0 to 6 months is 31 g/d, and 30 g/d for infants 7 to 12 months old. Otherwise, diet percentages are recommended for children (1–3 years old: 30%–40% of diet; 4–18 years old: 25%–35%) without specifying the number of grams per day.

Electrolyte and Micronutrient Needs

The provision of the correct balance of electrolytes, vitamins, minerals, and trace elements is essential in mitigating nutrition-related consequences. Micronutrients are critical to optimizing protein, fat, and carbohydrate utilization. Current guidelines for the addition of vitamins, minerals, and trace elements reflect the RDA and AI and are based on age and weight. Sodium, potassium, phosphorus, and magnesium are especially important for hydration and nitrogen balance.[66–68] Electrolyte management may be complicated by fluid shifts, existing deficiency, fluid loss through wounds or GI tract, increased insensible water loss, and renal failure.[44] Critically ill children often have severe phosphate and magnesium deficiency, and require repletion. Measurement from drained fluid may help in understanding repletion needs. In metabolic alkalosis from diuresis or suction of secretions from the GI tract, chloride administration should be considered to correct the pH.[44] For the critically ill child, if deficiencies exist supplementation is necessary. Although the ideal dose of micronutrients for sick children is unknown, a diet that includes required electrolytes and maximizes micronutrients to meet physiologic needs will promote recovery.[13]

ENTERAL NUTRITION

Enteral nutrition (EN) is the most common method of nutrition delivery in the PICU and is the recommended route of intake.[13] Enteral nutrition is associated with fewer clinical complications and alleviates a variety of nutrition-related concerns.[69] With EN the risk of translocation of the GI flora is limited, and intestinal integrity is preserved, preventing atrophy of the GI tract.[11]

Human Milk

Human milk is rich in the nutrients that support infant growth and development. A significant trait of human milk is the added bioavailability of nutrients in comparison with commercial infant formulas. Although standard infant formula provides adequate nutrition, human milk is preferred for all infants. The American Academy of Pediatrics (2012) recommends human milk for term, preterm, and other high-risk infants either by direct breastfeeding and or by expressed breast milk.[70]

The immunoglobulins available in human milk support a wide range of bacteriostatic and bactericidal activity, including boosting immunity against various GI infections. Additional nonnutrient components of human milk contribute to GI mucosal integrity and function.[71] Reducing untoward outcomes, including necrotizing enterocolitis, in preterm infants has been demonstrated.[71] Infants fed human milk also display a reduced incidence of celiac disease, inflammatory bowel disease, and obesity. Suboptimal breast feeding is also associated with acute lower respiratory infections in children younger than 5 years.[33] For infants whose mothers are unable to provide their own milk, donor milk is a suitable alternative for infants.[71] Maintaining appropriate equipment, space, and support for collection and storage of breast milk is necessary in all environments that care for critically ill infants.[72]

Commercial Enteral Formulas

When necessary, a commercial formula is selected based on the child's needs. A cow's milk or soy-based formula is typically adequate. The guiding principle in formula choice is usually composition of protein. Formula based on cow's milk contains lactose as the primary protein source, whereas soy-based formula contains soy protein. Standard infant formulas contain more calcium, phosphorus, and vitamin D than human milk, because absorption of these elements is limited in formula. In addition, most infant formulas contain approximately 40% to 50% fat. Infant and pediatric formulas vary in their concentration, with an increasing trend toward including both LCT and MCT oils. One advantage of medium-chain fatty acids is their ability to be absorbed directly into the bloodstream. For infants with additional difficulties with nutrient absorption, digestion, and transport, or severe intractable diarrhea, peptide-based formulas are available with hydrolyzed casein and MCT. Lactose-free formulas support digestion and absorption. Soy-based formulas may also be used for infants displaying signs of primary or secondary lactose intolerance. Special formulas are configured to support various other health conditions including prematurity and renal disease. For children with CHD a formula low in LCT and high in MCT is often preferred, because MCT does not increase chyle production in the lymphatic system.

Enhancement of human milk and infant formula are often necessary and beneficial for infants with critical illness. Increasing energy needs often necessitates an increase in caloric density from the standard 20 cal/oz to 24 or 27 cal/oz (and at times 30 cal/oz). By adding less water to formula powder, caloric density can be increased. Human milk fortifier is often used with breast milk to add calories. Single modular macronutrient components (protein, fat, or carbohydrate) can be added to commercially prepared formulas.[72] With manipulation of caloric density and changes in nutrient distribution, the increase in renal solute load must be considered.

Enteral products specifically designed for children 1 to 10 years of age first entered the market in the 1980s. In general, pediatric formulas provide a higher caloric value and are configured to meet the needs of this age group. Peptide-based formulas are used with increasing frequency in the pediatric population. Higher visceral protein levels have been demonstrated in patients receiving peptide-based formulas instead of those containing intact protein.

Adult formulations are considered safe for most children older than 10 years. Standard adult formulas necessitate normal digestive capacity. For those patients with malabsorption, predigested or elemental formulas reduce bile-acid excretion and require minimal digestion. These formulas contain oligopeptides or amino acids as protein and are usually hyperosmolar, making them more appropriate for older children and adolescents.

Fiber

Fiber also has a place in the enteral feeding plan. Pediatric formulas including fiber may benefit critically ill children with diarrhea, constipation, neuromuscular disease, and immobility. By reducing diarrhea, the child holds a better chance for nutrient absorption.[73–75] Fiber-enriched formulas are also commonly considered for patients receiving long-term enteral feeding. For patients at risk of bowel ischemia and severe dysmotility, fiber should be avoided.[73]

Enteral Nutrition Delivery

Delivery of enteral feedings can be accomplished by an intermittent or continuous method. Intermittent feedings mimic normal eating patterns and allow the gut to rest. Continuous feedings, however, are often preferred in the ICU setting. Starting with a small volume of full-strength formula is typically the most appropriate approach. Subsequent increases in volume should be based on patient tolerance. Diluting formula contributes to the delay in reaching nutritional goals, and should be avoided.[76]

The debate over the best EN delivery route persists. The route chosen depends on GI function, the expected duration of tube feeding, and the child's potential for aspiration. Feeding the child via the stomach allows gastric acid and other hormones to respond normally in the digestive process. Typically higher osmotic loads are tolerated in the stomach, with a lower incidence of dumping syndrome. Additional advantages of the gastric route include ease of tube placement and decreased cost. Because of the theoretical advantages, transpyloric tubes are often preferred for feeding the critically ill infant and child. Transpyloric feedings reduce interruptions and volume of gastric residuals.[77] Postpyloric feedings may also supply more calories compared with gastric feedings.[78] To some clinicians postpyloric enteral tube placement supports the value and safety of early nutrition, and is recommended when gastric feedings fail. A recent meta-analysis by a Chinese medical team yielded 15 randomized clinical trials that examined postpyloric versus gastric feeding, and found a reduction in pneumonia with postpyloric feeding.[79,80] The risk of aspiration and vomiting, however, were not significantly different between patients treated with gastric and postpyloric feeding. Other pediatric studies have demonstrated no efficacy in the use of postpyloric feeding in comparison with gastric feeding. In addition to aspiration, gastroesophageal reflux has been noted in children with transpyloric tubes, especially during periods of feeding. No difference in feeding tolerance, growth and development, and feeding-related complications were noted in transpyloric and gastric feedings for premature infants.[81] In addition, no difference in the incidence of diarrhea, vomiting, and GI motility has been observed between transpyloric and gastric feedings. For these reasons, ASPEN does not recommend a site of delivery of EN.[13]

Timing

For the average ICU patient, nutritional deficiencies build up over the first week of hospitalization. Infants are especially vulnerable because of their reduced energy stores and added risk of hyperglycemia. Although brief nutritional inadequacies may have limited consequences, if adequate oral intake is not expected within 24 to 48 hours of admission, alternative methods should be sought.[82] Early aggressive EN increases protein intake and improves protein balance during acute stress response.[44] Early feeding with small peptide-based protein improves nitrogen balance and returns prealbumin to normal levels.

In addition, early feeding mitigates the breakdown of glycogen and fat stores, and reduces the innate inflammatory response.[83,84] For patients with acute respiratory distress syndrome (ARDS), early feedings with trophic amounts in comparison with full feedings have the same effect on ventilator-free days, infectious complications, and mortality at 60 days.[85] In a meta-analysis of early enteral feedings the results suggest an overall treatment effect consistent with a large reduction in mortality and infectious complications.[86] In particular, trauma patients appear to have a decrease in mortality with early feedings.[87]

Gaps in Prescription and Delivery

Achieving the nutrient delivery goal is a consistent issue for ICU patients.[88] Children in PICUs often to not receive satisfactory caloric intake despite the amount prescribed.[20] DeGroof and colleagues[89] noted that only 25% of children with meningococcal sepsis achieved their goal.

ASPEN acknowledges that barriers exist to adequate EN delivery.[13] Providing nutrition during the early and the most critical stages of illness is often challenged by fluid restriction, operative and procedural interruptions, worries of feeding intolerance, and functional issues such as displaced or clogged feeding tubes.[90,91] In addition, use of catecholamines interferes with advancement of feedings and achievement of adequate calories.[21] In addition, when health care workers identify feeding intolerance (58% of patients), a 1-day median interruption occurs.[91]

Strategies are needed to identify and prevent avoidable delays in nutrition therapy. A nutrition support team and predicable advancement protocols positively affect nutrient delivery in critically ill patients. Gurgieora and colleagues[92] demonstrated that the EN rate increased from 25% to 60% with the implementation of a nutrition support team.

Management of residuals varies, especially in children, and affects interruptions and, therefore, EN delivery.[91] Gastric residual volume (GRV) is not a surrogate for aspiration related to gastric emptying. Although there is no evidence to support the acceptable or unacceptable volume, some suggest that a GRV of 5 mL/kg or 150 mL is significant.[13] With repeated measurement (every 2 hours), EN can be held and monitored for 4 hours and then restarted at 50% of previously fed volume.

The use of vasopressors alone is also not a contraindication to feed the gut. However, caution is needed for those children on inotropes that have strong α-agonist activities. These α-agonists may affect ischemia and increase the likelihood of bowel injury.[62]

Enteral Complications and Limitations

Enteral feeding is not complication free. Intolerance of EN may be indicated by ileus, abdominal distention, and heme-positive stools.[62] EN is also associated with a risk of nosocomial pneumonia.[82,93] Although EN is preferred, those who receive EN alone often do not reach energy goals, and underfeeding with EN alone may increase mortality at 60 days.[81,94]

PARENTERAL NUTRITION

Parenteral nutrition (PN) is used in the PICU when the enteral route cannot be used or is unable to provide sufficient nutrients.[13] By administering nutrients directly into the bloodstream, PN can provide all the calories to maintain prescribed amounts. In a multicenter cohort study of nutrition practices in 31 PICUs from 8 countries, PN provided nutrition exclusively to 8.8% of patients and in combination with EN to 21% of patients.[28] With the addition of PN, energy balance was more likely to be achieved in this sample. This finding was supported by other investigators noting that those patients who receive PN either alone or in combination with EN were more likely to attain their goal energy intake.[20,95] A randomized trial and a meta-analysis found that PN adjusted to provide lower glucose concentrations (instead of hyperglycemic levels) is as reliable as EN in adult patients.[96] In addition, children who were malnourished and those who received PN had a higher chance of receiving satisfactory nutrition.[28]

According to Jeejeebhoy,[67] the use of PN depends on function of the GI tract and duration of feeding. The type and quantity of the nutrient fed may also influence the decision to use PN. In addition, the clinical condition of the child and its metabolic effect influence the urgency of PN. Conditions such as trauma, sepsis, renal failure, and hepatic failure influence the use and requirements for nutrients. Candidates for PN also include children with intractable vomiting/diarrhea, paralytic ileus, severe short bowel syndrome, graft versus host disease, and cystic fibrosis, and children following bowel resection. Many of these children have a dysfunctional GI tract and are unable to absorb nutrients, requiring a higher caloric intake than EN can provide.

Although there is agreement that initiation of PN is initiated in a step-by-step process, there continues to be a debate about when to start PN. ASPEN recommends PN after 7 days of hospitalization for the adult patient who is of normal nutrition status, whereas the European Society for Clinical Metabolism and Nutrition recommend 24 to 48 hours if normal nutrition cannot be obtained in 2 to 3 days.[13,97] Mascarenhas and Wallace[98] recommend starting PN if the patient is nil by mouth (NPO) for more than 3 days for the malnourished child, and in the well-nourished child if NPO longer than 5 days. For the trauma patient it may be necessary to begin feeding within the first 3 days from injury.[62] Most experts concur that patients with short lengths of stay, especially when they demonstrate adequate growth and development, should not be prioritized for PN.[99]

Before beginning PN, caloric needs are estimated and daily fluid requirements are calculated based on patient attributes. Fluids can be altered for those with high insensible losses, and decreased for those who need less fluid. Although standard commercial preparations are available, PN is often tailored to the critically ill child's nutritional needs and metabolic status. PN typically requires 5% to 10% fewer calories than enteral requirements because of the thermic effect of food absorption.

Protein is administered in the form of crystalline amino acids. Amino acids maintain nitrogen balance even in the absence of adequate caloric intake in malnourished patients.[67,100] Each gram of protein contains 4 kcal, and up to 20% and no less than 10% of calories are recommended. Infant and preterm solutions contain cysteine, histamine, tyrosine, and taurine. The low pH of PN allows additional calcium and higher amounts of branch-chain amino acids to be added.[98] In addition, amino acid preparations are available with a nutrient configuration most suited for children with renal disease and hepatic encephalopathy.

The amount of protein in PN is calculated by using body weight and multiplying by estimated protein needs for age and condition. In pediatric patients with bronchiolitis, those given 3.1 g/kg/d demonstrated a positive protein balance whereas those receiving 1.7 g/k/d did not.[67] There may be greater protein needs for sick patients who have sepsis, protein-losing enteropathy, and malnutrition. Higher protein amounts improve survival in pediatric burns patients.[63]

The remaining calories in PN are divided between carbohydrates and fat.[98] Targeting carbohydrate calories to 50% to 60% is common, with dextrose providing 3.4 cal/mL. The concentration of dextrose should be prescribed while keeping in mind the need to avoid hyperglycemia and hypercapnia. Standard lipid administration as part of a parenteral diet recommends 25% to 35% fat with a maximum of 60%.

The addition of lipids to meet energy targets decreases the amount of glucose infused, thereby reducing the risk of hyperglycemia and use of insulin to normalize serum glucose.[67] Lipid emulsions are triglycerides with egg phospholipids containing glycerol, which is added to render the solution isotonic. These emulsions can be a combination of LCT and MCT. In the United States, Intralipids contain only LCT. These standard fat emulsions contain linoleic acid with omega-6 fatty acids dominating the concentration of omega-3 fatty acids. Omega-6 fatty acid is a precursor of proinflammatory prostaglandins and thromboxanes, and should be infused at controlled rates. In Europe several formulations are available with both MCT and LCT. Fat emulsions are provided in a 20% solution (2.2 kcal/L). An initial rate of 1 g/kg/d is safe. Advancement can be safely done by monitoring triglycerides. Maximum lipid dose is 3 g/kg/d. If the triglycerides level is higher than 400, one should consider halving the lipid dose.

The pediatric multivitamin solution added to PN includes vitamin K, lower amounts of B vitamins, and larger amounts of vitamin D. The adult formulation for children older than 11 years contains appropriate levels of calcium and phosphorus for age, and no vitamin K. PN routinely includes zinc, iron, copper, chromium, manganese, and selenium. For those with liver disease the amount of copper can be decreased to 50%, whereas an increase in copper is recommended for those children with burns.[98] Decreasing manganese in those patients with hepatobiliary disease has also been recommended.[12] When bicarbonate levels are running low, sodium acetate can be added to PN.

The peripheral route can be used for children with normal fluid requirements and an expected need for calories for no longer than 1 week. Glucose concentration limits peripheral administration, and an osmolarity of less than 1000 osmol/L is recommended.[98] An increase in the child's basic fluids may be necessary to achieve good distribution of macronutrients.

While on PN, robust laboratory monitoring should occur. It is recommended always to check electrolytes to obtain a baseline measurement before starting PN. Initially electrolytes as well as calcium, magnesium, and phosphorus should be checked daily and then liberalized as patient status and PN stability is achieved. Adjustments in PN can then be made based on routine analysis of serum levels.

PN differs from EN in safety and efficacy. Overfeeding and a prolonged hypercaloric state are of particular concern with PN because of the ease of adding calories to these artificial solutions. A 2012 investigation noted that PN was associated with a higher mortality in PICU patients. In addition, a recent multisite clinical trial of adult patients found that PN started at less than 48 hours from admission (rather than after day 8 of admission) resulted in more infectious complications and a prolonged length of stay.[64] Kutsogiannis and colleagues[101] found that use of PN was associated with patients experiencing ARDS and those who had longer lengths of hospital stay before admission to the ICU. Metabolic complications, such as hyperglycemia, and technical issues involving catheter displacement and breakage can also occur with PN. Sepsis risk seems to be a continuing issue despite some investigators questioning study methodology, and speculation that the relationship to infection may be that of hyperglycemia and lack of protein rather than PN.[67] Nonetheless, when PN is optimized to an adequate delivery of calories a neutral caloric balance results, and achieves a dramatic effect on mortality and morbidity.[97]

SUMMARY

A child's added energy requirements and lower macronutrient stores combined with the stress of illness make the critically ill infant and child less able to withstand nutritional deprivation. Newborns are especially at risk for poor nutritional status during an ICU stay. Conventional nutrition for critically ill infants and children requires a diet specific to their needs with a mix of macronutrients. For children with significant metabolic demands, the quantity of nutrients can be manipulated. Administering protein in itself has an important influence on immune function including wound healing. Prior nutrition status and severity of the current illness assist in determining the initiation of nutritional support. Matching nutrient prescription with delivery affects nutrition outcomes. Clinical response to feeding is the best indicator of nutritional adequacy. The potential effect of undernutrition on an already compromised child must lead the health care team to ensure the child's nutritional needs are addressed early in their PICU stay.

REFERENCES

1. Alberda C, Gramlich L, Jones N, et al. The relationship between nutritional intake and clinical outcome in critically ill patients: results of an international multicenter observation study. Intensive Care Med 2009;35:1728–35.

2. Bistrian BR, Blackburn GL, Vitale J, et al. Prevalence of malnutrition in general medical patients. Am J Clin Nutr 1974;32:1320–5.
3. Hendricks KM, Duggan C, Gallagher L, et al. Malnutrition in hospital pediatric patients: current prevalence. Arch Pediatr Adolesc Med 1995;149:1118–22.
4. Heyland D. Critical care nutrition support research: lessons learned from recent trials. Curr Opin Clin Nutr Metab Care 2013;16:176–81.
5. Merritt RJ, Suskind RM. Nutritional survey of hospitalized pediatric patients. Am J Clin Nutr 1929;32:1320–5.
6. Schetz M, Casaer M, Van den Bergh G. Does artificial nutrition improve outcome of critical illness? Crit Care 2013;17:302.
7. Pichard C, Kyle UG, Morabia A, et al. Nutritional assessment: lean body mass depletion at hospital admission is associated with an increased length of stay. Am J Clin Nutr 2004;79:613–8.
8. Bechard L, Parrott JS, Mehta N. Systematic review of the influence of energy and protein intake on protein balance in critically ill children. J Pediatr 2012; 161:333–9.
9. de Betue CT, Waardenburg DA, Deutz NE, et al. Increased protein-energy intake promotes anabolism in critically ill infants with viral bronchiolitis: a double-blind randomized controlled trial. Arch Dis Child 2011;96:817–22.
10. McClave SA, Heyland D. The physiologic response and associated clinical benefits from provision of early enteral nutrition. Nutr Clin Pract 2009;24:305–15.
11. Heyland DK, Chalill N, Day AG. Optimal amounts of calories for critically ill patients: depends on how you slice the cake. Crit Care Med 2011;38:2619–36.
12. Kirkland LL, Kashiwagi DT, Brantley S, et al. Nutrition in the hospitalized patient. J Hosp Med 2013;8:52–8.
13. Mehta NM, Compher C. ASPEN clinical guidelines: nutrition support of the critically ill child. JPEN J Parenter Eternal Nutr 2009;33:260–76.
14. Seike J, Tangoku A, Yuasa Y, et al. The effect of nutritional support on the immune function in the acute postoperative period after esophageal cancer surgery: total parenteral nutrition versus enteral nutrition. J Med Invest 2011;58: 75–80.
15. Heyland DK, Dhaliwal R, Drover JW, et al, Canadian Critical Care Clinical Practice Guidelines Committee. Canadian clinical practice guidelines for nutrition support in mechanically ventilated, critically ill adult patients. JPEN J Parenter Eternal Nutr 2003;7:355–73.
16. Botran M, Lopez-Herce J, Mencia S, et al. Enteral nutrition in the critically ill child: comparison of standard and protein-enriched diets. J Pediatr 2011;159: 27–32.
17. Briassoulis G, Filippou O, Hatzi E, et al. Early enteral administration of immunonutrition in critically ill children: results of a blinded randomized controlled clinical trial. Nutrition 2005;21:799–807.
18. van Waardenburg DA, de Betue CT, Goudoever JB, et al. Critically ill infants benefit from early administration of protein and energy-enriched formula: a randomized controlled trial. Clin Nutr 2009;28:249–55.
19. Martin CM, Doig GS, Heyland DK, et al, Southwestern Ontario Critical Care Research Network. Multicentre, cluster-randomized clinical trial of algorithms for critical-care enteral and parenteral therapy (ACCEPT). CMAJ 2004;170: 197–204.
20. de Menezes FS, Leite HP, Koch PC, et al. What are the factors that influence the attainment of satisfactory energy intake in pediatric intensive care unit patients receiving enteral or parenteral nutrition? Nutrition 2013;29:76–80.

21. de Neef M, Geukers VG, Dral A, et al. Nutritional goals, prescription and delivery in a pediatric intensive care unit. Clin Nutr 2008;27:65–71.
22. Giner M, Laviano A, Meguid MM, et al. In 1995 a correlation between malnutrition and poor outcome in critically ill patients still exists. Nutrition 1996;12: 23–9.
23. Hulst J, Joosten K, Zimmermann L, et al. Malnutrition in critically ill children: from admission to 6 months after discharge. Clin Nutr 2004;23:223–32.
24. Kuzu MA, Terzioglu H, Gene V, et al. Preoperative nutritional risk assessment in predicting postoperative outcome in patients undergoing major surgery. World J Surg 2006;30:378–90.
25. Pollack M, Wiley JS, Kanter R, et al. Malnutrition in critically ill infants and children. JPEN J Parenter Eternal Nutr 1982;6:20–4.
26. Pollack M, Ruttimann UE, Wiley J. Nutritional depletion in CIC: association with physiologic instability and increased quality of care. JPEN J Parenter Eternal Nutr 1985;9:309–13.
27. Sungurtekin H, Sungurtekin U, Oner O, et al. Nutrition assessment in critically ill patients. Nutr Clin Pract 2008;23:635–64.
28. Mehta NM, Bechard LJ, Chahill N, et al. Nutrition practices and their relationship to clinical outcomes in critically ill children-an international multicenter cohort study. Crit Care Med 2012;40:2204–11.
29. Heyland D, Schroter-Noppe D, Drover J, et al. Nutrition in the critical care setting current practice in Canadian ICUs—opportunity for improvement. JPEN J Parenter Eternal Nutr 2003;27:74–83.
30. Mentec H, Dupont H, Bocchetti M, et al. Upper digestive intolerance during enteral nutrition in critically ill patients: frequency, risk factors, and complications. Crit Care Med 2001;29:1955–61.
31. Reintam A, Parm P, Kitus R, et al. Gastrointestinal symptoms in intensive care patients. Acta Anaesthesiol Scand 2009;53:318–24.
32. Hiesmayr M. Nutrition risk assessment in the ICU. Curr Opin Clin Nutr Metab Care 2012;15:180.
33. Grant C, Wall C, Gibbons M, et al. Child nutrition and lower respiratory tract disease burden in New Zealand: a global context for a national perspective. J Paediatr Child Health 2011;47:497–504.
34. Correia MI, Waitzberg DL. The impact of malnutrition on morbidity, mortality, length of hospital stay and costs evaluated through a multivariate model analysis. Clin Nutr 2003;22:235–9.
35. Reilly JJ Jr, Hull SF, Albert N, et al. Economic impact of malnutrition: a model system for hospitalized patients. JPEN J Parenter Eternal Nutr 1988;12:371–6.
36. Medoff-Cooper B, Ravishankar C. Nutrition and growth in congenital heart disease: a challenge for children. Curr Opin Cardiol 2013;28:122–9.
37. Brinksma A, Huizinga G, Sulkers E, et al. Malnutrition in childhood cancer patients: a review on its prevalence and possible causes. Crit Rev Oncol Hematol 2012;83:249–75.
38. Sullivan PB, Lambert B, Rose M, et al. Prevalence and severity of feeding and nutritional problems in children with neurological impairment: Oxford Feeding Study. Dev Med Child Neurol 2000;42:674–80.
39. Martinez-Biarge M, Diez Sebastian J, Wusthoff CJ, et al. Feeding and communication impairments in infants with central grey matter lesions following perinatal hypoxic-ischaemic injury. Eur J Paediatr Neurol 2012;16:688–96.
40. Shaw S, Jaksic T. The metabolic needs of critically ill children and neonates. Semin Pediatr Surg 1999;8:131–9.

41. Joint Commission on Accreditation of Healthcare Organizations. Comprehensive accreditation for hospitals. Chicago: Joint Commission on Accreditation for Healthcare Organizations; 2007.

42. Food and Nutrition Board, Institute of Medicine of the National Academies. Dietary reference intakes for energy, carbohydrates, fiber, fat, fatty acids, cholesterol, proteins and amino acids. Washington, DC: National Academy press; 2005. Available at: http://books.nap.edu/openbook.php?record_id=10490. Accessed October 15, 2013.

43. Lee LW, Yan AC. Skin manifestations of nutritional deficiency disease in children: modern day contexts. Int J Dermatol 2012;51:1407–18.

44. Metha N, Duggan C. Nutritional deficiencies during critical illness. Pediatr Clin North Am 2009;56:1143–60.

45. Schneider SM, Veyres P, Pivot X, et al. Malnutrition is an independent factor associated with nosocomial infections. Br J Nutr 2004;92:105–11.

46. Waitzberg DL, Correia TD. Nutritional assessment in the hospitalized patient. Curr Opin Clin Nutr Metab Care 2003;6:531–8.

47. Mei Z, Grummer-Strawn LM, Pietrobelli A, et al. Validity of body mass index compared with other body-composition screening indexes for the assessment of body fatness in children and adolescents. Am J Clin Nutr 2002;75:7597–985.

48. Centers for Disease Control and Prevention Growth Charts. Available at: http://www.cdc.gov/growthcharts/. Accessed October 5, 2013.

49. Hulst JM, van Goudoever JB, Zimmermann LJ, et al. The effect of cumulative energy and protein deficiency on anthropometric parameters in the pediatric ICU population. Clin Nutr 2004;23(6):1381–9.

50. Fuhrman MP, Charney P, Mueller CM. Hepatic proteins and nutrition assessment. J Am Diet Assoc 2004;104:1258–64.

51. Selby A, Schell D. Indirect calorimetry in mechanically ventilated children: a new technique that overcomes the problem of endotracheal tube leak. Crit Care Med 1995;23:365–78.

52. Scholfield W. Predicting basal metabolic rate, new standards and review of previous work. Hum Nutr Clin Nutr 1985;39(Suppl 1):5–41.

53. Briassoulis G, Venkataramon J, Thompson AE, et al. Energy expenditure in critically ill children. Crit Care Med 2000;28:1166–72.

54. Coss-Bu JA, Jefferson L, Valding D, et al. Resting energy expenditure and nitrogen balance in critically ill pediatric paediatric patients on mechanical ventilation. Nutrition 1998;9:649–52.

55. Derumcoax-Burel H, Meyer M, Morn L, et al. Prediction of resting energy expenditure in a large population of obese children. Am J Clin Nutr 2004;80:1544–5.

56. Hardy CM, Dwyer J, Smelling LK, et al. Pitfalls in predicting RE requirement in critically ill child: a comparison of predictive methods to indirect calorimetry. Nutr Clin Pract 2002;17:182–9.

57. White M, Shepard R, McEniery J. Energy expenditure in 100 ventilated CIC improving the accuracy of predication equations. Crit Care Med 2000;28:2307–12.

58. Vazquez Martinez JL, Martinez Romillo PD, Diez Sebastian J, et al. Predicted versus measured energy expenditure by continuous online IC in ventilated CIC during early postoperative period. Pediatr Crit Care Med 2004;5:19–27.

59. Chwals W. Overfeeding the critically ill child: fact or fantasy? New Horiz 1994;2:147–55.

60. Singer P, Pichard C. Reconciling divergent results of the latest parenteral nutrition studies in the ICU. Curr Opin Clin Nutr Metab Care 2013;16:187–93.
61. Food and Nutrition Board of the Institutes of Health, National Academy of Sciences nutrient recommendations: dietary reference intakes (DRI). Available at: http://ods.od.nih.gov/Health_Information/Dietary_Reference_Intakes.aspx. Accessed October 10, 2013.
62. Cook RC, Blinman TA. Nutritional support of the pediatric trauma patient. Semin Pediatr Surg 2010;19:242–51.
63. Chan M, Chan G. Nutrition therapy for burns in children and adults. Nutrition 2009;25:261–9.
64. Casaer MP, Mesotten D, Hermans G, et al. Early versus late parenteral nutrition in critically ill adults. N Engl J Med 2011;37:506–17.
65. Wischmeyer P. Parenteral nutrition and calorie delivery in the ICU: controversy, clarity or call to action? Curr Opin Crit Care 2012;18:164–73.
66. Freeman JB, Wittin M, Stegink L, et al. Effects of magnesium infusions on magnesium and nitrogen balance during parenteral nutrition. Can J Surg 1982;25:570–2.
67. Jeejeebhoy KN. Parenteral nutrition in the intensive care unit. Nutr Rev 2012;70:623–30.
68. Rudman D, Millikan NJ, Richardson TJ, et al. Elemental balances during intravenous hyperalimentation of underweight adult subjects. J Clin Invest 1975;5:94–104.
69. Zamberlan P, Figueiredo Delgand A, Leone C, et al. Nutrition therapy in the PICU: implications, monitoring complications. JPEN J Parenter Eternal Nutr 2011;35:523–9.
70. American Academy of Pediatrics Section on Breastfeeding. Breastfeeding and the use of human milk (policy statement). Pediatrics 2012;115:496.
71. Ramani M, Ambalavanan N. Feeding practices and necrotizing enterocolitis. Clin Perinatol 2013;40:1–10.
72. Verger J, Lebet R, editors. AACN's Pediatric procedure manual for acute and critical care. Philadelphia: Elsevier; 2008.
73. Hayes GL, McKinzie BP, Bullington WM, et al. Nutritional supplements in critical illness. AACN Adv Crit Care 2011;22:301–16.
74. Spapen H, Diltoer M, Van Malderen C, et al. Soluble fiber reduces incidence of diarrhea in septic patients receiving total enteral nutrition: a prospective double-blind randomized and controlled trial. Clin Nutr 2001;20:301–5.
75. Weisen P, Van Gossum A, Preiser JC. Diarrhea in critically ill. Curr Opin Crit Care 2006;12:149–54.
76. Marshall AP, West SH. Enteral feeding in the critically ill: are nursing practices contributing to hypocaloric feeding? Intensive Crit Care Nurs 2006;22:95–105.
77. Montejo JC, Gau T, Acosta J, et al. Nutrition and metabolic working group of the Spanish Society of Intensive Care Medicine and Coronary Units. Multicenter, prospective randomized single blind study comparing the efficacy and GI complications of earl jejunal feeding with early gastric feeding in critically ill patient. Crit Care Med 1992;30:796–800.
78. Must A, Anderson SE. Effects of obesity on morbidity in children and adolescents. Nutr Clin Care 2003;6:4–12.
79. Meert KL, Daphtary KM, Metheny NA. Gastric versus small-bowel feeding in critically ill children receiving mechanical ventilation: a randomized controlled trial. Chest 2004;126:872–8.
80. Watson J, McGuire W. Transpyloric versus gastric tube feeding in premature infants. Cochrane Database Syst Rev 2013;(2):CD003487.

81. McClave SA, Sexton LK, Spain DA, et al. Enteral tube feeding in the intensive care unit: factors impeding adequate delivery. Crit Care Med 1999;27:1252–6.

82. Canadian Critical Care Clinical Practice Guidelines Committee. Canadian clinical practice guidelines for nutrition support in mechanically ventilated, critically ill adult patients. JPEN J Parenter Eternal Nutr 2003;27:355–73.

83. Moore EE, Jones TN. Benefits of immediate jejunostomy feeding after major abdominal trauma—a prospective randomized study. J Trauma 1986;26: 874–81.

84. Perel P, Yanagawa T, Bunn F, et al. Nutrition support for head injured patients. Cochrane Database Syst Rev 2006;(18):CD0001530.

85. The National Heart Lung and Blood Institute ARDS Clinical Trails Network. Initial trophic versus full enteral feedings in patient with acute lung injury. The EDEN Randomized Trial. JAMA 2012;307:795–803.

86. Early versus delayed EN clinical practice guidelines. Available at: http://www/criticalcarenutrition.com/index.php?option-com_content&view=category&layout=blog&id=21&1temid=10. Accessed September 25, 2013.

87. Doig GS, Huges P, Simpson F, et al. Early enteral nutrition reduces mortality in trauma patients requiring intensive care: a metanalysis of randomized control trials. Injury 2011;42:50–6.

88. Cahill NE, Heyland DK. Bridging the guideline-practice gap in critical care nutrition: a review of guideline implementation studies. JPEN J Parenter Eternal Nutr 2010;36:653–9.

89. deGroof F, Joosten KR, Janssen JA, et al. Acute stress response in children with meningococcal sepsis: important differences in growth hormone/insulin-like growth factor I axis between nonsurvivors and survivors. J Clin Endocrinol Metab 2002;87:3118–24.

90. Iglesias S, Liete H, Santonae Meneses J, et al. Enteral nutrition in critically ill children: are prescription and delivery according to their energy requirements? Nutr Clin Pract 2007;22:233–9.

91. Rogers EJ, Gilbertson HR, Heine RG, et al. Barriers to adequate nutrition in critically ill children. Nutrition 2003;19:865–8.

92. Gurgieora G, Lieke HR, Tadder JA, et al. Outcomes and PICC before and after implementation of nutrition support team. JPEN J Parenter Eternal Nutr 2005;29: 176–85.

93. Jiyong J, Tiancha H, Huiqin W, et al. Effect of gastric versus post-pyloric feeding on the incidence of pneumonia in critically ill patients: observations from traditional and Bayesian random-effects meta-analysis. Clin Nutr 2013;32:8–15.

94. Adam S, Batson S. A study of problems associated with the delivery of enteral feed in critically ill patients in five ICUs in the UK. Intensive Care Med 1997;23: 261–6.

95. Oosterveld MJS, van der Kuip M, de Meer K, et al. Energy expenditure and balance following pediatric intensive care unit admission: a longitudinal study of critically ill children. Pediatr Crit Care Med 2006;7:147–53.

96. Simpson F, Doig GS. Parenteral vs. enteral nutrition in the critically ill patient: a meta-analysis of trials using the intention to treat principle. Intensive Care Med 2005;31:12–23.

97. Singer P, Berger MM, Van den Berghe G, et al. ESPEN guidelines on parenteral nutrition: intensive care. Clin Nutr 2009;28:387–400.

98. Mascarenhas M, Wallace E. Parenteral nutrition. In: Willier R, Hyams J, Kay M, editors. Pediatric gastroenterology and liver disease. 4th edition. Philadelphia: Elsevier; 2012.

99. de Aguilar-Nascimento J, Bicudo-Salomao A, Portari-Filho P. Optimal timing for the initiation of enteral and parenteral nutrition in critical medical and surgical conditions. Nutrition 2012;28:840–3.
100. Greenberg GR, Jeejeebhoy KN. Intravenous protein-sparing therapy in patients with gastrointestinal disease. JPEN J Parenter Eternal Nutr 1979;3:427–32.
101. Kutsogiannis L, Alberda C, Gramlich L, et al. Early use of supplemental parenteral nutrition in critically ill patients: results of an international multicenter observational study. Crit Care Med 2011;39:2691–9.

Nutrition in the Chronically Ill Critical Care Patient

Marthe J. Moseley, PhD, RN, MSN, CCNS[a,b,*]

KEYWORDS

- Chronic critical illness • Clinical practice nutrition guidelines • Adult critical care
- Nutritional risk

KEY POINTS

- Chronically critically ill adult patients are at risk for suboptimal outcomes.
- Clinical practice nutrition guidelines provide recommendations and evidence to optimally support critically ill patients at risk for compromise.
- Critical care nurses need to have an understanding of the guidelines as well as other forms of research evidence to guide critical care teams in planning interventions for patients.

INTRODUCTION

Survival from critical illness is due in large part to advances in critical care. This new population of patients (survivors of critical illness), however, will ultimately require further care and are referred to as chronically critically ill. Critically ill patients are at particular risk of malnutrition, which occurs in up to 40% of critical care cases. Chronic critical illness includes those patients with persistent respiratory failure, dysfunction of organ systems, presence of complications of pressure ulcers, and infections as well as other conditions imposing burdens on patients at each subsequent critical care admission. Critical illness in any patient with chronic disease presents problems when planning care, especially when the preexisting condition of alteration in nutritional status is present. The purpose of this article is to give recommendations for care to the chronically critically ill patient population in need of nutrition optimization.

ASPEN GUIDELINES

The American Society for Parenteral and Enteral Nutrition (ASPEN) has published guidelines for nutrition screening, assessment, and intervention in critically ill adults.

Disclosure Statement: The author discloses that she is a representative on the Nursing Advisory Board for Elsevier/MC Strategies.
[a] Office of Nursing Services, Veterans Healthcare Administration, Washington, DC, USA;
[b] Rocky Mountain University of Health Professions, Provo, UT, USA
* 101 Bikeway Lane, San Antonio, TX 78231.
E-mail address: Marthe@satx.rr.com

These guidelines are used in the practice setting to provide critical care nurses with evidence to influence decision making. Decision making based on solid evidence optimizes care planning to meet expected outcomes in chronically critically ill patients. Guideline recommendations allow critical care nurses to associate the use of published recommendations for nutrition screening and assessment to the anticipated clinical outcomes. The impact of the nutrition assessment and supported interventions on patient outcomes is considered in the context of nutrition status.[1] Published guidelines and written recommendations for care are often assigned a specific level of evidence. **Table 1** gives an example of leveling of evidence with the description assigned to each level. In addition, recommendations may be given a grading (**Table 2**). An aid in understanding the strength of the evidence published to support the recommendations[1] is thinking of this as giving a report card to the recommendation. The information gleaned from **Table 1** is used to interpret the descriptions listed in **Table 2**. Three interventions and practices from the ASPEN guidelines are initially recommended for consideration in caring for chronically critically ill patients with nutrition alterations (**Table 3**). Note the grades of these recommendations (E and C). The first 2 recommendations are supported by level IV or V evidence and the third recommendation is supported by at least one level II investigation.

IMPLEMENTING RISK ASSESSMENT INTO PRACTICE

The benefits of implementing guideline recommendations include improved screening, detection, and monitoring of patients at risk for malnutrition as well as planning for improvement in nutrition status. On admission to a critical care unit, a critical care nurse initiates the admission assessment, including the screen for nutrition risk. For anyone at risk for malnutrition or currently malnourished, interventions are initiated by a critical care team to address the alterations identified from the assessment data. There are several tools available to determine risk in critically ill patients. The subjective global assessment (SGA) was used to evaluate a prospective cohort of 309 patients with renal failure to predict severe undernutrition in 42% of patients.[2] SGA identifies malnutrition, distinguishes malnutrition from a disease state, predicts outcome, and identifies patients in whom nutritional therapy can alter outcome. The novel risk assessment tool is a validated scoring method quantifying nutrition risk in critically ill patients.[3] The study had a total of 597 patients were enrolled in this prospective, observational study of patients expected to stay greater than 24 hours. As a score increased in the multivariable model, so did mortality rate and duration of mechanical ventilation.

Table 1	
Levels of evidence and description	
#	**Description**
I	Large randomized trials with clear-cut results; low risk of false-positive (α) and/or false-negative (β) error
II	Small, randomized trials with uncertain results; moderate to high risk of false-positive (α) and/or false-negative (β) error
III	Nonrandomized cohort with contemporaneous controls
IV	Nonrandomized cohort with historical controls
V	Case series, uncontrolled studies, and expert opinion

Data from Academy of Nutrition and Dietetics. Critical illness evidence-based nutrition practice guideline. Chicago: Academy of Nutrition and Dietetics; 2012.

Table 2	
Strength of evidence recommendation and description	
Grade of Evidence Recommendation	**Description**
A	Supported by at least two level I investigations
B	Supported by one level I investigation
C	Supported by at least one level II investigation
D	Supported by at least one level III investigation
E	Supported by level IV or V evidence

Data from Academy of Nutrition and Dietetics. Critical illness evidence-based nutrition practice guideline. Chicago: Academy of Nutrition and Dietetics; 2012.

There are several screening tools that have been developed to assess for nutritional risk in different patient populations.[4] The Nutritional Risk Index has been used in surgical patients using serum albumin and percentage of usual body weight to stratify nutritional risk. The SGA is used for both the surgical and oncology patient populations and the Mini Nutritional Assessment has applicability in all general geriatric populations. There is not, however, a screening tool validated in the chronically critically ill.

EVIDENCE FOR USE OF ENTERAL NUTRITION

After completion of risk assessment and subsequent identification of chronically critically ill patients, critical care nurses consider additional nutrition recommendations.[5] The next important recommendation is that enteral nutrition is recommended over parenteral nutrition support. Contraindications to enteral nutrition include hemodynamic instability, bowel obstruction, high-output fistula, and/or severe ileus. Research has shown less septic morbidity, fewer infectious complications, and cost savings in enteral fed critically ill adults compared with parenteral fed adults in the critical care environment.[5]

Every practice guideline has the potential to reference a different set of criteria for the rating scheme regarding the strength of the evidence as well as the strength of the recommendation. The critical illness evidence-based nutrition practice guideline[5] uses a grading system based on updates by the American Dietetics Association (ADA) Research Committee to an existing system whereby the strength of the grade (I–V) is assigned a descriptive of good/strong, fair, limited/weak, expert opinion only, or grade not assignable. The most beneficial portion of this type of rating is noted within the

Table 3		
Recommendations for nursing interventions and practice and grade		
#	**Recommendations**	**Grade of Recommendation**
1.	Screening for nutrition risk is suggested for hospitalized patients.	E
2.	Nutritional assessment is suggested for all patients who are identified to be at nutrition risk by nutrition screening.	E
3.	Nutrition support intervention is recommended for patients identified by screening and assessment as at risk for malnutrition or malnourished.	C

Data from Mueller C, Compher C, Druyan ME, American Society for Parenteral and Enteral Nutrition (A.S.P.E.N.) Board of Directors. A.S.P.E.N. clinical guidelines: nutrition screening, assessment, and intervention in adults. JPEN J Parenter Enteral Nutr 2011;35(1):16–24.

implication for practice section. A statement rating of strong means that a recommendation is followed unless clear and compelling rationale is present. A fair statement rating implies that the recommendation is generally followed; however, critical care nurses are to remain alert to new evidence and patient preferences. A weak recommendation implies caution for critical care nurses in deciding whether to follow the recommendation, exercising judgment and being alert if new evidence emerges. A consensus recommendation or expert opinion implies flexibility of the critical care nurse in implementing the recommendation, especially in the face of patient preference. Finally, insufficient evidence implies that critical care nurses use constraint to follow the recommendation.

The recommendations taken from this guideline include the descriptive grade and the statement label (conditional vs imperative). Conditional statements define a specific situation whereas imperative statements are broadly applicable to the target population. The first recommendation is that enteral nutrition is started within 24 to 48 hours of admission to the critical care environment.[5–7] This is a strong recommendation with a conditional evidence statement label. An example of use of this recommendation is that if a critical care nurse is assigned a chronically critically ill patient admitted 8 hours prior, then tube feedings should be started. A second recommendation is that if a critically ill adult is on a ventilator, then a small-bore feeding tube is placed for feeding. Research studies suggest that small bowel enteral nutrition versus gastric enteral nutrition reduces ventilator-associated pneumonia.[5] This is a fair recommendation with a conditional statement label. Another recommendation is that when feeding a critically ill patient, at least 60% of the total estimated energy requirement should be received as enteral nutrition within the first week of hospitalization, because this is associated with fewer infectious complications.[5,6] This recommendation statement is described as fair and has an imperative statement label.

Practical recommendations in enterally fed critically ill patients cover an array of intervention areas.[5] For example, blue dye is not used in the feedings to evaluate for aspiration, because the risk of using blue dye outweighs any perceived benefit of using it. The recommendation is fair and contains an imperative statement label. Another recommendation is that the head of bed elevation for critically ill patients is placed at 30° to 45° to promote a decrease in the incidence of aspiration pneumonia and reflux of gastric contents into the esophagus and pharynx. The recommendation is strong with an imperative statement label. The next recommendation is that in the absence of signs of intolerance (**Box 1**) in critically ill patients, gastric residual volumes of less than 500 mL are not a reason for holding enteral nutrition. The recommendation is fair with a conditional statement label. Strong, conditional evidence indicates that when 200 to 500 mL of gastric residual volumes exist, promotility agents are used.

EVIDENCE FOR MONITORING OF GASTRIC RESIDUAL VOLUME

There are practice recommendations specific to the monitoring of gastric residual volumes, which are described in greater detail.[5] The clinical practice guideline specific to

---

Box 1
Indicators of intolerance

- Abdominal distention
- Nausea
- Vomiting

the monitoring of enteral nutrition (**Table 4**) actually assigns a grade to the level of evidence. This type of scale is used for this set of recommendations assigning a grade of A when good research-based evidence supports the recommendation, for example, a prospective, randomized trial was located for evidence. A grade of B is assigned when there are fair research-based recommendations to support the guideline; for example, a well-designed study without randomization was found to provide evidence for this recommendation. And, finally, a grade of C is assigned when the guideline recommendation is based on expert opinion and/or editorial consensus. Eight recommendations are provided with associated levels of evidence for the monitoring of gastric residual volume in critically ill patients.

EVIDENCE OF RECOMMENDATIONS FOR ENTERAL NUTRITION IN CRITICALLY ILL

In 2 different summaries,[8,9] recommendations for enteral nutrition in critically ill patients were based on the most widely used guidelines of different scientific societies specific to the use of enteral nutrition in critically ill patients. The levels of evidence in these examples use a different scoring. This source is according to the GRADE Working Group. These recommendations are included in **Table 5**.

CHRONIC DISEASE CONSIDERATIONS

Some specific chronic disease states require special considerations for enteral nutrition. **Table 6** lists specific disease states, including renal failure, liver failure, pancreatitis, respiratory failure, abdominal surgery, and cardiac disease. Each of these disease states includes corresponding considerations for intervention relative to these

Table 4
Monitoring of gastric residual volume

Recommendation	Level of Evidence
Evaluate all enterally fed patients for risk of aspiration.	A
Assure that the feeding tube is in the proper position before initiating feedings.	A
Keep the head of the bed elevated at 30°–45° at all times during the administration of enteral feedings.	A
When possible, use a large-bore sump tube for the first 1–2 d of enteral feeding and evaluate GRV using at least a 60-mL syringe.	A
Check GRV every 4 h during the first 48 h for gastrically fed patients after enteral feeding goal rate is achieved and/or the sump tube is replaced with a soft, small-bore feeding tube; GRV monitoring may be decreased to every 6–8 h in noncritically ill patients.	C
Every-4-h measurements, however, are prudent in critically ill patients.	B
If the GRV is ≥250 mL after a second GRV check, a promotility agent should be considered in adult patients.	A
A GRV >500 mL should result in holding enteral nutrition and reassessing patient tolerance by use of an established algorithm, including physical assessment, gastrointestinal assessment, evaluation of glycemic control, minimization of sedation, and consideration of promotility agent.	B
Consideration of a feeding tube placed below the ligament of Treitz when GRVs are consistently measured at >500 mL.	B

Abbreviation: GRV, gastric residual volume.
Data from Academy of Nutrition and Dietetics. Critical illness evidence-based nutrition practice guideline. Chicago: Academy of Nutrition and Dietetics; 2012.

Table 5
Summary of recommendations with assigned level of evidence for enteral nutrition in critically ill patients

Summary of Recommendations for Enteral Nutrition in Critically Ill Patients	Level of Evidence
Enteral nutrition is associated with an improvement of nutritional variables, a lower incidence of infections and a reduced length of hospital stay.	A (consistent level 1 studies)
Critically ill patients who cannot be fed orally for a period of more than 3 d must receive specialized nutritional support.	C (level 4 studies or extrapolations from level 2 or 3 studies)
Enteral nutrition is preferable to parenteral nutrition.	B (consistent level 2 or 3 studies or extrapolations from level 1 studies)
Enteral nutrition should be started within the first 24–48 h of admission.	A (consistent level 1 studies)
Enteral nutrition should provide 25–30 kcal/kg/d.	C (level 4 studies or extrapolations from level 2 or 3 studies)
The feedings should be advanced toward goal over the next 48–72 h.	C (level 4 studies or extrapolations from level 2 or 3 studies)
The enteral nutrition must be deferred until the patient is hemodynamically stable.	C (level 4 studies or extrapolations from level 2 or 3 studies)
In intensive care unit patients, neither the presence nor absence of bowel sounds and evidence of passage of flatus and stool is required for initiation of enteral nutrition.	B (consistent level 2 or 3 studies or extrapolations from level 1 studies)

Data from Hegazi R, Wischmeyer P. Clinical review: optimizing enteral nutrition for critically ill patients – a simple data-driven formula. Crit Care 2011;15:234; 1–11; and Seron-Arbeloa C, Zamora-Elson M, Labarta-Monzon L, et al. Enteral nutrition in critical care. J Clin Med Res 2013;5(1):1–11.

chronic illness states.[8] These considerations are important for critical care nurses in planning optimal nutrition support outcomes.

NUTRITION SUPPORT TEAM AND SPECIAL CONSIDERATIONS

Not only do critical care nurses need to stay on top of any change in nutritional status in chronically critically ill patients but also a nutrition support team must be notified of ongoing progress toward meeting goals the team has mutually set. A nutrition support team service was studied to determine effect on critical care patient outcomes.[13] Nutrition supply type and patient outcomes were retrospectively analyzed in those patients who received either parenteral or enteral nutrition support during their stay. Those who received the benefit of the team support realized a reduction in the length of hospital stay, reduction in the average days of fasting, decreased number of days on parenteral nutrition (equating to cost savings), and increased number of calories delivered to enhance adequate nutrition support.

Special considerations require specific team members' expertise to deliver optimal nutrition support. Careful evaluation is considered regarding the use of immune-modulating enteral nutrition in critically ill patients without acute respiratory distress syndrome (ARDS) or acute lung injury (ALI).[5] There has been fair, conditional status on the recommendations because some mixed populations have shown benefit in reduction of infection complications. In patients with ARDS or ALI, there is strong

Table 6
Chronic illness states and corresponding considerations

Chronic Disease State	Considerations
Renal failure[8]	Preserve lean mass and energy reserves Avoid malnutrition Attenuate the inflammatory response and oxidative stress Improve endothelial function Monitor serum electrolytes (phosphorus, potassium, and magnesium) Monitor micronutrient levels (zinc, selenium, thiamin, folic acid, and vitamins A, C, and D)
Liver failure[8]	Caloric intake of 25–40 kcal/kg/d with mixed energy substrates (carbohydrates and fats) Branched-chain amino acids enriched diet not recommended Increased vitamins and trace elements
Pancreatitis[8]	Enteral feedings into the jejunum within first 48 h Maintain minimum enteral nutrient supply
Respiratory failure	Protein supply 1.0–1.8 g/kg/d[8] High-fat, low-carbohydrate formulas not indicated[8] Attend to potassium, phosphorus, magnesium, and antioxidants[8] Enrich with omega-3 fatty acids[8] Avoid calorie overload[10] Address nutrition issues[11]
Abdominal surgery[8]	Early postoperative enteral feeding Use of omega-3 fatty acids and glutamine supplementation in surgical patients receiving parenteral nutritional support
Cardiac disease[12]	Monitor for cardiac cachexia resulting from chronic congestive heart failure and malnutrition due to complications postoperative cardiac surgery Sustained hyperglycemia in the first 24-h post–acute coronary syndrome has a poor prognostic factor for 30-d mortality Support nutritional state with 20–25 kcal/kg/d Protein intake 1.2–1.5 g/kg/d Restrict sodium and volume according to patient clinical situation Major energy source for myocytes is glutamine through conversion to glutamate (protective of myocardial cells from ischemia) Omega-3 1 g/d supplement in the form of fish oil

conditional evidence to consider using immune-modulating enteral formulas with fish oil, borage oil, and antioxidants. Fair, imperative data exist that supplemental glutamine is not recommended for routine use.

Calorie delivery to critically ill patients is considered of cardinal importance.[14] Adequate nutrition has distinct effects on immune function and inflammatory pathways and in these conditions is associated with increased morbidity impairing survival.[8] Patients ventilated on either pressure or volume control modes of ventilation were studied while infusing insulin to maintain a target blood glucose level.[14] All of the subjects received enteral or parenteral feeding as part of their standard treatment. Findings suggested that energy requirements were met in only 24% of the feeding days, accounting for a discrepancy between caloric prescription and intake caused by underfeeding in nearly half of critical care patients and overfeeding in 27% of the study days, leading to the conclusion that nutritional care of critically ill patients is complicated.

Special considerations take into account specific recommendations for blood glucose levels in that they are kept less than 180 mg/dL.[15] Yet in chronically critically ill patients, intensive metabolic support with control of intensive insulin therapy, early and consistent nutrition support, and nutritional pharmacology advance knowledge for this very sick population of patients.[4] Research needs in the critically ill discuss the optimal management of chronically critically ill patients to include nutrition and glucose control.[16]

Initiation of therapy requires consideration. There is a significant association between severity of illness and timing of enteral feeding initiation[17]; 108 critically ill patients were studied in a retrospective observational study grouped as less severe and more severe. One group of patients received enteral feeding within 48 hours of admission. Feedings beginning after this time frame were assessed as late feeding cases. Among patients who were more severely ill yet early feeders, improved nutritional outcomes were realized, claiming nutrition as a beneficial option.

A randomized multicenter trial was conducted to compare early initiation of parenteral nutrition with late initiation in adults in critical care when nutrition targets could not be met by enteral nutrition alone.[18] In 2312 patients, parenteral nutrition was initiated less than 48 hours after admission to a critical care unit. In 2328 patients, the parenteral nutrition was not started before the eighth day. Both groups had early enteral nutrition started as well as insulin infusion to target normal glycemic control. The subjects in the late initiation group had an increased likelihood of 6.3% of being discharged alive earlier from the critical care environment and from the hospital without evidence of decreased functional status at hospital discharge. In addition, the late initiation group had fewer ICU infections and lower incidence of cholestasis.

Surgical critically ill patients also have unique considerations for nutrition care. Perioperative use of glutamine in patients at risk of moderate to severe malnutrition before surgery is an effective option for decreasing morbidity associated with malnutrition.[19] Glutamine therapy improves blood glucose modulation and reduces infection and critical care unit stay. Glutamine depletion was demonstrated to be an independent predictor of hospital mortality in critically ill patients.[20] The prevalence of glutamine and glutathione depletion was performed in an observational study relating to mortality and the conventional predictors of mortality outcome. The admission plasma glutamine concentrations were independent of the conventional risk scoring at admittance, and a subnormal concentration was an independent predictor of mortality.

A question was posed regarding knowledge enhancement in those with chronic illness supposing that education regarding maintaining nutritional health could be influenced. A systematic review was completed to evaluate interventions to improve health literacy for chronic disease.[21] One of the subsets of behavioral risk factors for change included nutrition. The Cochrane Library, Joanna Briggs Institute, Medline, Embase, CINAHL, PsychINFO, Web of Science, Scopus, APAIS, Australasian Medical Index, Google Scholar, Community of Science, and 4 targeted journals were searched resulting in 52 studies selected for inclusion. Interventions for groups and the individual in the community settings were more effective in supporting sustained nutrition change than interventions in primary health care. Effective interventions may target multiple behaviors without compromising effectiveness.

Other studies of special consideration have been undertaken. A prospective study of a cohort of chronically critically ill patients was conducted to determine how often advance directives and appropriate surrogates were available to guide decisions about life-sustaining treatments, including nutrition therapy.[22] Most patients had poor clinical outcomes, with more than two-thirds of the 230 patients experiencing a major complication during the treatment of chronic critical illness, half of whom were ventilator dependent. Among the 5 therapies under study, nutrition and hydration along with mechanical ventilation were least often limited. The median time to limitation of nutrition was almost 3 weeks. In this cohort, renal replacement therapy and vasopressors were limited more often. The view that food and water must always be offered has deep cultural and/or religious roots. Thus, in this study, decisions to limit treatment were not made proactively, based on balancing of expected burdens and benefits. Instead decisions were deferred until the last days of a prolonged and complicated hospital course, when patients were already close to death. Clarification of patient and family goals, values, and objectives assist to influence decisions to limit life-sustaining treatment. Treatment clarification is coupled with conscious health care decisions informed by effective communication.

Chronic critical illness is an important problem in the care of patients with nutrition alterations. The ultimate goal for chronic critical illness is liberation from mechanical ventilation, leading to improved survival and enhanced quality of life. In the face of an acute critical care admission, any of the chronic disease states may find treatment options inclusive of mechanical ventilation therapy. Optimizing the chronic critical illness strategies of weaning off the ventilator requires meticulous attention to metabolic and nutritional parameters.[4]

SUMMARY

Chronic critical illness is a problem in the critical care environment. The ultimate goals in managing care for the chronically critically ill are early enteral feeding and liberation from mechanical ventilation, leading to improved survival and enhanced quality of life. Clinical practice guidelines and evidence to support the recommendations in the guidelines are presented as a framework in providing care for this distinct patient population. Research studies supplement the recommendations to ensure best care guides critical care decisions using the best available evidence in the context of patient values and clinical expertise.

REFERENCES

1. Mueller C, Compher C, Druyan ME, American Society for Parenteral and Enteral Nutrition (A.S.P.E.N.) Board of Directors. A.S.P.E.N. clinical guidelines: nutrition screening, assessment, and intervention in adults. JPEN J Parenter Enteral Nutr 2011;35(1):16–24.
2. Cano N, Aparicio M, Brunori G, et al. ESPEN guidelines on parenteral nutrition: adult renal failure. Clin Nutr 2009;28:401–14.
3. Heyland D, Dhaliqal R, Jiang X, et al. Identifying critically ill patients who benefit the most from nutrition therapy: the development and initial validation of a novel risk assessment tool. Crit Care 2011;15:R268, 1–11.
4. Schulman R, Mechanick J. Metabolic and nutrition support in the chronic critical illness syndrome. Respir Care 2012;57:958–78.
5. Academy of Nutrition and Dietetics. Critical illness evidence-based nutrition practice guideline. Chicago: Academy of Nutrition and Dietetics; 2012.
6. Dellinger RP, Levy MM, Rhodes A, et al, Surviving Sepsis Campaign Guidelines Committee including the Pediatric Subgroup. Surviving sepsis campaign: international guidelines for management of severe sepsis and septic shock: 2012. Crit Care Med 2013;41(2):580–637.
7. Bankhead R, Boullata J, Brantley S, et al. A.S.P.E.N. enteral nutrition practice recommendations (Monitoring enteral nutrition administration). JPEN J Parenter Enteral Nutr 2009;33(2):162–6. (Special Report).
8. Seron-Arbeloa C, Zamora-Elson M, Labarta-Monzon L, et al. Enteral nutrition in critical care. J Clin Med Res 2013;5(1):1–11.

9. Hegazi R, Wischmeyer P. Clinical review: optimizing enteral nutrition for critically ill patients – a simple data-driven formula. Crit Care 2011;15(234):1–11.

10. Grau Carmona T, Lopez Martinez J, Vila Garcia B. Guidelines for specialized nutritional and metabolic support in the critically-ill patient. Update. Consensus SEMICYUC-SENPE: respiratory failure. Nutr Hosp 2011;26(Suppl 2):37–40.

11. Criner G, Cordova F, Sternberg A, et al. The national emphysema treatment trial (NETT): Part 1: lessons learned about emphysema. Am J Respir Crit Care Med 2011;184:763–70.

12. Jimenez Jimenez F, Cervera Montes M, Blesa Malpica A. Guidelines for specialized nutritional and metabolic support in the critically-ill patient. Update. Consensus SEMICYUC-SENPE: cardiac patient. Nutr Hosp 2011;26(Suppl 2): 76–80.

13. Mo Y, Rhee J, Lee E. Effects of nutrition support team services on outcomes in ICU patients. Yakugaku Zasshi 2011;131(12):1827–33.

14. De Waele E, Spaen H, Honore P, et al. Bedside calculation of energy expenditure does not guarantee adequate caloric prescription in long-term mechanically ventilated critically ill patients: a quality control study. ScientificWorldJournal 2012;909564:1–6.

15. Department of Veteran Affairs, Department of Defense. VA/DoD clinical practice guideline for the management of diabetes mellitus. Washington, DC: Department of Veteran Affairs, Department of Defense; 2010. p. 146.

16. Carson S. Research needs and strategies to establish best practices and cost effective models for chronic critical illness. Respir Care 2012;57(6):1014–8.

17. Huang H, Hsu C, Kang M, et al. Association between illness severity and timing of initial enteral feeding in critically ill patients: a retrospective observational study. Nutr J 2012;11:30.

18. Casaer M, Mesotten D, Hermans G, et al. Early versus late parenteral nutrition in critically ill adults. N Engl J Med 2011;365:506–17.

19. Orfila G, Talaveron J. Effectiveness of perioperative glutamine in parenteral nutrition in patients at risk of moderate to severe malnutrition. Nutr Hosp 2011;26(6): 1305–12.

20. Rodas P, Rooyackers O, Hebert C, et al. Glutamine and glutathione at ICU admission in relation to outcome. Clin Sci (Lond) 2012;122:591–7.

21. Taggart J, Williams A, Dennis S, et al. A systematic review of interventions in primary care to improve health literacy for chronic disease behavioral risk factors. BMC Fam Pract 2012;13:49.

22. Camhi S, Meracado A, Morrison S, et al. Deciding in the dark: advance directives and continuation of treatment in chronic critical illness. Crit Care Med 2009;37(3): 919–25.

Malnutrition in the ICU Patient Population

Jan Powers, PhD, RN, CCRN, CCNS, CNRN*, Karen Samaan, PharmD, BCNSP

KEYWORDS

- Malnutrition • Critically ill patients • Enteral nutrition • Parenteral nutrition
- Specialized nutrition

KEY POINTS

- Hospitalized patients entering the intensive care unit (ICU) are at a significantly increased risk for malnutrition.
- Nutritional therapy should be initiated within 24 to 48 hours of admission to the ICU.
- Enteral nutrition is the preferred route of administration for nutritional therapy in the patient in the ICU.

INTRODUCTION

Critically ill or injured patients are a diverse group with diagnosis ranging from a planned surgery or respiratory failure secondary to community-acquired pneumonia, to multiple bone trauma or serious burns. Each patient represents a different level of care; however, all are at risk for inflammation. Inflammation has been associated with malnutrition and malnutrition has been associated with compromised immune status, infection, and increased intensive care unit (ICU) and hospital length of stay (LOS). Some critically ill patients may present to the ICU with a known risk or diagnosis of malnutrition; however, many will present well nourished, but quickly develop inflammatory-induced acute malnutrition. Therefore, it is imperative that all critically ill patients are screened for nutritional needs and nutrition therapy initiated once the patient is stabilized, ideally within the first 24 to 48 hours of admission.

CRITICAL ILLNESS AND MALNUTRITION

Malnutrition is commonly viewed as a chronic condition due to lack of food or nutrients secondary to environmental, social, or psychological etiologies. It has been identified

Disclosure Statement: J. Powers is on the speaker's bureau for Abbott Nutrition and Sage Medical Products. She has also received research support from Corpak Medsystems and Sage Medical Products. K. Samaan has no disclosures to report.
St. Vincent Hospital, 2001 West 86th Street, Indianapolis, IN 46260, USA
* Corresponding author. St. Vincent Hospital, 2001 West 86th Street, Indianapolis, IN 46260.
E-mail address: jmpowers@stvincent.org

as a cause for disease as well as a condition resulting from acute and chronic disease or inflammation.[1] Malnutrition is common in acute-care settings, occurring in 30% to 50% of hospitalized patients[2-6] and has been associated with decreased organ function, abnormal laboratory values,[6] longer hospital LOS,[3] increased falls,[4,5] increased incidence of pressure ulcers, and significantly increased mortality.[3] Somanchi and colleagues[6] found a reduced LOS by identifying malnutrition and offering nutrition intervention early in hospitalized patients.

During critical illness, several factors affect the loss of lean body mass: previous functional status or lean body mass, severity of critical illness/injury, intensity of the inflammatory response, restoration of physiologic enteral nutrition (EN), and balance between protein breakdown and protein synthesis.[1,7-13] Varying degrees of acute and/or chronic inflammation are key factors in pathogenesis of malnutrition in critically ill or injured patients. The presence of inflammation also promotes anorexia and blunts the effectiveness of nutrition strategies.[1,9,11,12] The catabolism of muscle may be self-limiting as the critical illness resolves; however, if it is sustained, it will contribute to increased morbidity and poor outcomes.[1,11]

The acute inflammatory response promotes cytokine-driven protein catabolism of skeletal muscle and increases energy and protein demands.[1,14] Endogenous nutrient utilization is mediated by the counter-regulatory hormones, including epinephrine, cortisol, glucagon, and growth hormone, which oppose the anabolic effects of insulin. Although insulin is often readily available during inflammation, skeletal muscle and other end organs are often resistant to its effect. This response occurs rapidly and only normalizes after the acute insult resolves; therefore, early nutrition assessment and delivery are warranted.[1,7,10,15-20]

MALNUTRITION DEFINED

Over the past decade, malnutrition in hospitalized patients has been given close attention following mandates from the Joint Commission for nutrition screening within the first 24 hours of admission. In 2009, only 3% of adult hospital admissions in the United States included a diagnosis of malnutrition.[10] Reports in the literature are as high as 60%; this discrepancy has been attributed to variability of "definitions" for malnutrition, nutrition assessment tools, and criteria used for assessment, and disease state variability.[1,7,10,11]

In 2009, an International Guideline Committee, including the American Society for Parenteral and Enteral Nutrition[12] (A.S.P.E.N.) and European Society for Clinical Nutrition and Metabolics,[1] developed and published an etiology-based approach to the diagnosis of adult malnutrition syndromes in acutely ill patients (**Table 1**). This approach includes the evaluation of the presence of inflammation and delineates whether malnutrition is related to starvation, chronic disease, acute illness, or injury. It is important to note that patients could have one or more of these syndromes simultaneously and can also transition from one to another.[1]

These recommendations were followed by a consensus statement in 2012 by the Academy of Nutrition and Dietetics and the A.S.P.E.N. consensus statement recommending standardized characteristics for the identification and documentation of adult malnutrition.[7,10] Although the statement focused on undernutrition, the investigators stated that "overweight and obese patients experiencing critical illness or injury are at risk for malnutrition and benefit from the same nutrition intervention as other critically ill patients." Undernutrition was used synonymously with malnutrition and was described as a lack of adequate calories, protein, or other nutrients needed for tissue maintenance and repair occurring along a continuum of

Table 1		
Malnutrition syndromes proposed by an International Guideline Committee including A.S.P.E.N. and European Society for Clinical Nutrition and Metabolics include the recognition of acute systematic inflammatory response		
Starvation-Associated Malnutrition	Chronic Disease–Associated Malnutrition	Acute Disease– or Injury-Associated Malnutrition
Chronic starvation without inflammation	Mild to moderate degree chronic inflammation	Severe degree acute inflammation
Anorexia nervosa, depression, alcoholism, poverty	Pulmonary disease, cancer, rheumatoid arthritis, sarcopenia	Major infection, burns, trauma, closed head injury

Data from Jensen GL, Mirtallo J, Copher C, et al. Adult starvation and disease-related malnutrition: a proposal for etiology-based diagnosis in the clinical practice setting from the International Consensus Guideline Committee. Clin Nutr 2010;291:151–3.

inadequate intake, impaired absorption, and altered utilization and transport of nutrients.[10]

The groups agreed that adults meeting at least 2 of 6 identified characteristics (**Box 1**) would meet diagnostic criteria for malnutrition. The investigators provided a tool that further distinguished between severe and nonsevere malnutrition. Assessment of these characteristics is recommended at admission and throughout patient care, including acute, transitional, and chronic care, as the etiology and severity of malnutrition may change along with caloric requirements and nutrient needs.[10]

SCREENING AND ASSESSMENT

Early screening of nutritional status in critically ill patients will help identify patients at nutritional risk and facilitate the initiation of nutrition therapy.[10,11,13,15] Patients with identified needs will benefit from early nutritional interventions. It is reasonable to consider any patient staying for 2 or more days in the ICU without normal oral intake at risk for malnutrition.[9]

Box 1	
Adults meeting at least 2 of 6 identified characteristics meet diagnostic criteria for malnutrition	

Criteria for the Identification and Documentation of Adult Malnutrition

1. Insufficient energy intake

2. Weight loss

3. Loss of muscle mass

4. Loss of subcutaneous fat

5. Localized or generalized fluid accumulation that may sometimes mask weight loss

6. Diminished functional status as measured by hand-grip strength

Data from White JV, Guenter P, Jensen G, et al, The Academy Malnutrition Work Group, the A.S.P.E.N. Malnutrition Task Force, the A.S.P.E.N. Board of Directors. Consensus statement: Academy of Nutrition and Dietetics and American Society for Parenteral and Enteral Nutrition: Characteristics Recommended for the Identification and Documentation of Adult Malnutrition (Undernutrition). JPEN J Parenter Enteral Nutr 2012;36(3):275–83.

When screening, identification of chronic conditions at admission is key, as these represent a chronic inflammatory state with possible preexisting malnutrition.[10,11] Evaluating the patient's acute conditions for risk of inflammation and the characteristics of malnutrition helps identify and diagnose simultaneous malnutrition syndromes or increased severity of preexisting malnutrition. Examples of chronic disease states include pulmonary disease, alcohol abuse, and cancer. Of note, advanced age, poverty, and dementia greatly increase a patient's risk for undernutrition. A body mass index (BMI) less than 25 or 35 or higher has been associated with greater benefit of early, aggressive nutritional therapy.[19]

Many risk assessment screening tools are available, but there is no ICU-specific scoring system including nutrition-related indicators.[7,9] Using the disease-related malnutrition syndromes and characteristics described in **Table 1** and **Box 1** will help identify risks and diagnose disease-related malnutrition. In addition, clinical signs of inflammation should be assessed, such as fever, hypothermia, and tachycardia.

After the initial screen for malnutrition, a more in-depth nutrition assessment is performed. This is typically completed by a registered dietician. Nutrition history includes 3 key indicators: actual weight (admission) and height for calculation of the BMI, history of recent weight loss (past 3–6 months), and recent decrease in nutrient intake.[9] Laboratory indicators are not helpful, as there are no tests that allow for diagnosis of malnutrition. Traditionally, low circulating levels of albumin and prealbumin have been used to identify malnutrition; however, these carrier proteins are used during the inflammatory response for cytokine delivery into tissue and, therefore, low circulating levels are more indicative of an inflammatory response versus nutritional status.[13,15]

NUTRITION THERAPY

Nutrition in the critical care setting has evolved from a supportive role with goals of maintaining lean body mass and immune function while preventing metabolic complications to a more focused therapeutic role aimed to minimize the metabolic response to inflammation and evade disease-related malnutrition.[13,18] Nutrition therapy includes early EN, appropriate macronutrient and micronutrient delivery, avoiding overfeeding and underfeeding, and glycemic control.[13,21]

Estimating Energy Needs

When providing nutritional therapy, it is important to first determine the caloric goal and needs of the patient. Indirect calorimetry is considered the "gold standard" for determining energy needs; however, this technique has limitations, including the need for stable conditions, and is time consuming and expensive.[22] Most ICUs do not have access to indirect calorimetry, and use predictive equations to estimate energy needs. There are many predictive equations available; however, none have been shown to correlate with indirect calorimetry measurements in critically ill patients.[7,22] In addition to predictive equations, the American College of Chest Physicians recommends 25 kcal/kg per day[23] and A.S.P.E.N. gives caloric estimates of 25 to 30 kcal/kg per day for moderately stressed patients (surgical, critical care) and 30 to 35 kcal/kg per day for severely stressed patients (trauma, burns, sepsis).[17]

In the past, nutrition prescriptions did not include protein calories. It was thought protein would be spared if calories were provided through carbohydrate and fat sources. Complications of nutrition were thought to be secondary to glucose overload, but research found it was all the components of the nutrition prescription and overfeeding in general.[7,18,19,24] Overfeeding calories proved to have poor outcomes, including carbon dioxide retention with more days on the ventilator, hyperglycemia and impaired wound healing, and hepatic steatosis.[7,19,24–26] The use of "total calories," including calories from all sources, was adopted by nutrition practitioners.[25]

Due to the catabolic state, protein plays a significant role in nutrition therapy of the critically ill patient. Depending on the patient's condition, protein requirements vary from 1.4 to 2.5 g/kg per day based on level of stress, type of injury, and/or comorbidities.[13,27,28] Metabolic demands fluctuate over the hospital course as the patient's severity of illness and healing process dictate. Patients with severe injuries can increase their resting energy requirements by 100% or more.[29] Providing adequate calories to meet these high demands can be challenging.

Most recent attention has been given to energy requirements in the critical care setting after several trials have resulted in conflicting results regarding decreased calorie delivery on ventilator days, ICU/hospital LOS, and mortality.[18,19,30,31] These studies surround underfeeding patients (permissive underfeeding or trophic feeding), resulting in decreased ventilator days and mortality and those involving cumulative caloric deficits associated with increased ICU/hospital LOS and mortality. Caloric deficits contributed to delayed initiation of nutrition therapy, EN intolerance, and interruption of enteral feeding for procedures. These results led to investigations of supplementing inadequate EN delivery with parenteral nutrition (PN) to meet measured or estimated energy needs. These trials have reported conflicting results as well.[7,19,32–35] Each had its own limitations, which collectively have highlighted the need to deliver adequate initial protein to all patients; consider individual energy needs based on preexisting illness, severity of disease, and risk for mortality; and, finally, assess and adjust caloric requirements on a frequent basis. Well-organized randomized controlled trials (RCTs) are necessary to evaluate energy requirements and outcomes in the critically ill patient. Despite the controversy regarding optimal energy needs, it is agreed that early nutrition therapy is indicated in critically ill patients.[13,15,16]

Delivery of Nutritional Support

Some non–mechanically ventilated ICU patients can receive oral nutrition; however, it has been demonstrated that patients allowed oral diets consumed only 52% of estimated energy requirements.[22] Inadequacy of oral intake has been defined as less than 75% of daily requirements.[36]

Most ICU patients are unable to receive nutrients via the oral route and require specialized nutrition. Evidence-based practice guidelines strongly support EN over PN whenever possible.[13,15] When compared with PN, EN consistently reduces infectious morbidity and is associated with decreased hospital LOS.[13,15] PN is more costly, not only with regard to the nutrition admixture, but also the cost of venous access.

National and international guidelines support starting early EN for ICU patients within 24 to 48 hours of ICU admission when hemodynamically stable.[13,15] During critical illness, adverse changes to gut integrity and functionality result in an impaired immune response associated with an increased risk for systemic infection and multisystem organ dysfunction syndrome.[13] EN maintains the functional and structural integrity of the gastrointestinal (GI) tract through stimulation of the villi and supports the gut and mucosal immunity. Early EN is intended to maintain gut integrity, modify stress and the systemic immune response, and minimize disease severity.[13]

The most common access to the GI tract for delivery of EN in patients in the ICU is gastric, via a nasogastric or orogastric tube. This affords the most normal route of nutrition, but it is not without potential complications. These complications include nausea, vomiting, delayed gastric emptying, diarrhea, constipation, and abdominal cramping.[37] Caloric deficits can occur due to multiple interruptions, especially early in therapy. These interruptions result in cumulative caloric deficits and malnutrition; in fact, most critically ill patients receiving EN, average only 49% to 70% of their caloric goal.[15,35–40]

Gastric feedings require adequate GI tract motility and gastric emptying. Impaired GI motility and delayed gastric emptying are common in critically ill patients because of immobility, fluid imbalances, electrolyte disturbances, and medications (**Table 2**).[40–44] Similar to symptoms associated with other GI tract problems, symptoms of delayed gastric emptying include nausea, vomiting, abdominal distension, and bloating. When feeding the stomach, intolerance raises the concern for aspiration and pneumonia. In addition to physical assessment, gastric residual volumes (GRVs) are often measured and monitored to assess gastric emptying. Of note, there is no clear evidence that GRVs are related to the incidence of aspiration pneumonia.[13] A.S.P.E.N and the Society of Critical Care Medicine (SCCM) Guidelines for the Provision and Assessment of Nutrition Support Therapy in the Adult Critically Ill Patient

Table 2		
Fluid and electrolyte disorders and medications affecting GI motility		
Fluid Imbalance	**Electrolyte Disorders**	**Medications**
Dehydration can result in intravascular volume depletion leading to splanchnic hypoperfusion and potential bowel ischemia	Hypokalemia • Potassium needed for neuromuscular function associated with GI motility • Severe hypokalemia can result in paralytic ileus	Opioid Analgesics (eg, morphine, fentanyl, dilaudid) GI opioid receptors regulate motility and secretion Transit time is increased and pancreatic and intestinal secretions are inhibited Dose and duration of therapy contribute to constipation
Overhydration can lead to bowel edema and impaired response to gut hormones and neurotransmitters contributing to GI dysmotility and nutrient malabsorption	Hypomagnesemia • Magnesium is needed for neuromuscular function associated with GI motility • Hypomagnesemia contributes to hypokalemia	Catecholamines (eg, norepinephrine, dopamine) Vasopressors support blood pressure after fluid resuscitation. These patients are at risk for GI hypoperfusion and hypoxia and the adrenergic response may add to decreased GI motility and enteral nutrition intolerance
		Alpha-2 adrenergic receptor agonists (dexmedatomidine, clonidine) Thought to bind to receptors in the intestine and promote sodium and water absorption from the intestine, leading to altered GI function Clonidine is used to decrease high ostomy output Animal studies suggest dexmedetomidine inhibits gastric and ileal transit time

Abbreviation: GI, gastrointestinal.
Data from Btaiche IF, Lingtak-Neander C, Pleva M, et al. Critical illness, gastrointestinal complications, and medications therapy during enteral feeding in critically ill adult patients. Nutr Clin Pract 2010;25:32–49.

state that holding EN for GRVs to less than 500 mL in the absence of other signs of intolerance should be avoided.[13] For GRVs of 200 to 500 mL, guidelines recommend that aspiration pneumonia precautions are taken.[13] These include raising the head of the bed 30 to 45 degrees, continuous feeding, initiating a prokinetic agent when appropriate, and consideration of postpyloric feeding (**Table 3**).

Postpyloric or small bowel feedings are indicated in patients who do not tolerate gastric feedings, are at a risk of aspiration, are post major abdominal surgery, or have active pancreatitis. In a recent meta-analysis of 17 RCTs comparing gastric to postpyloric feedings, it was found that postpyloric feeding delivered more calories and helped reduce the GRV.[45] However, there was no difference in aspiration, new-onset pneumonia, or mortality.[45]

Parenteral Nutrition

In the critical care setting, PN is reserved for malnourished patients and those at nutritional risk, when EN is not possible. Complications of PN include those that are mechanical, metabolic, and infectious; therefore, the benefits of its use must be weighed against the risks. According to critical care guidelines, hemodynamically stable, malnourished patients without access to the enteral route or functioning GI tract are candidates for early PN.[13,15] Other patients considered for PN include massive small-bowel resection, proximal high-output fistulae, perforated small bowel, bowel obstruction, and severe GI bleeding.[13,46] It is recommended that PN be initiated when EN is not tolerated or contraindicated for more than 5 to 7 days. Well-nourished patients who are expected to receive EN or oral nutrition within 7 days of admission are not considered candidates.[13]

PN can be administered through a peripheral or central vein. Because the peripheral route delivers minimal protein calories and has a risk of phlebitis because of the admixture's high osmolality, it is typically not used and the central route is preferred.[46] It is important to maintain the sterility of the central line during PN administration to

Table 3	
Steps to reduce the risk of aspiration pneumonia	
Switch gastric bolus feedings to continuous feeding	Large-volume bolus feeding has been linked to increased incidence of aspiration pneumonia and reduced energy intake
Elevate head of bed 30°–45°	Compared with patients in the supine or semirecumbent position, elevating the head of the bed reduced the incidence of pneumonia
Initiate a prokinetic agent when GRV >200 mL	Metoclopramide and erythromycin improve gastric emptying and tolerance to enteral nutrition.
Initiate oral opioid antagonist therapy	Naloxone administered through enteral tubes has been shown to reverse the effects of narcotics on the GI tract and improved GI motility. It has been associated with improved energy intake and reduced GRV
Consider postpyloric tube placement when gastric residuals exceed 500 mL	Changing enteral feeding from the stomach to the small bowel reduces the incidence of regurgitation and aspiration

Abbreviations: GI, gastrointestinal; GRV, gastric residual volume.
Data from McClave SA, A.S.P.E.N. Board of Directors, American College of Critical Care Medicine. Guidelines for the Provision and Assessment of Nutrition Support Therapy in the Adult Critically Ill Patient: Society of Critical Care Medicine (SCCM) and American Society for Parenteral and Enteral Nutrition. JPEN J Parenter Enteral Nutr 2009;33:277–316.

minimize the risk for central line–related bloodstream infections (CLRBSI). It is imperative that health care professionals adhere to the guidelines for prevention of CLRBSI published by the Centers for Disease Control and Prevention for insertion and maintenance of central lines.[47]

PN is a complex sterile admixture of amino acids, dextrose, electrolytes, multivitamins, trace elements, and sometimes medications, such as insulin.[48] Intravenous fatty emulsion (IVFE) can be included in the PN admixture, known as a total nutrient admixture (or 3-in-1) or can be infused separately from the PN (2-in-1 admixture). Because compatibility of components within the admixture is dependent on pH, concentration of individual components, and temperature, it is important to inspect the 2-in-1 solutions for precipitation and the 3-in-1 solutions for lipid breakdown before administration. To avoid administration of particulates and microprecipitates, it is recommended to use a 1.2-μm filter for PN administration.[46] Because the contents of the PN admixture are a fine balance within itself, introducing another drug at the Y-site can introduce a possible interaction. It is recommended to use a different intravenous (IV) site for medication infusion unless the drug to be infused is documented as compatible with the PN formulation.[49]

Adjunctive therapies

The focus on nutrition and the immune system has brought attention to individual nutrients and their role in the immune and inflammatory response and cell protection.[8] Specific amino acids, omega-3 fatty acids, antioxidants, and prebiotics and probiotics have been studied in trauma, burn, and critically ill surgical patients.[8,14] **Table 4** lists these nutrients and their potential role in nutrition therapy. A number of EN formulas include some or all of these ingredients to modulate the immune response, attenuate inflammation, or improve wound healing in surgical, trauma, and burn patients; their place in nutrition therapy is controversial.[14]

COMMON COMPLICATIONS OF SPECIALIZED NUTRITION THERAPIES

Metabolic complications associated with nutrition therapy include fluid and electrolyte imbalances, hyperglycemia, azotemia, overfeeding-related complications, and PN-associated hypertriglyceridemia and liver abnormalities.[25,45] Patients in the critical care setting receive fluids from multiple sources, including maintenance fluids, intermittent intravenous piggy-back medications, tube feeding flushes for feeding tube maintenance, and medication administration and nutrition therapy. All patients, regardless of delivery of nutrition support, are at risk for fluid imbalance. Daily weights and strict documentation of intake and output are necessary to evaluate fluid status. Other indicators of fluid imbalance are serum sodium, blood urea nitrogen, blood pressure, and heart rate. Hyponatremia in a patient with weight gain and positive fluid balance may indicate fluid overload. Hypernatremia with azotemia in a patient with weight loss and a negative fluid balance suggests a possible fluid deficit. Dehydration is more likely to occur with EN, as it is a dense caloric source, whereas PN allows for liberal fluid administration. It is important to evaluate the patient's medications for use of diuretics, such as furosemide, which may impact fluid and electrolyte balance. Azotemia is also an indicator of protein intolerance, especially in patients with liver and renal dysfunction because of the inability to excrete urea.[25]

Electrolyte disturbances can occur with both EN and PN. Patients who are malnourished or with prolonged periods of NPO (nothing by mouth) are at particular risk for severe hypophosphatemia, hypokalemia, and hypomagnesemia. After a few days of starvation, in an effort to conserve somatic protein, the body shifts from glucose metabolism to fatty acid oxidation and uses ketones for energy.[9,50] When nutrition is

Table 4
Pharmaconutrients associated with immune response, anti-inflammation, and cellular protection

Pharmaconutrient	Role in Critical Illness	Recommendations and Cautions
Arginine Immune modulating Anti-inflammatory	• Arginine is conditionally essential during times of stress secondary to increased arginine metabolism • Arginine deficiency results in immune suppression	• In patients after major surgery, arginine combined with omega-3 fatty acids reduced infection and decrease length of stay when compared with standard formulas • Avoid in patients with severe sepsis. Arginine supplementation in patients with sepsis may worsen the inflammatory response and increase mortality
Omega-3 fatty acids Anti-inflammatory Cellular protection	• Systemic inflammatory response syndrome is a precursor to sepsis and multiorgan failure syndromes including ARDS and ALI • Omega-3 fatty acids can alter the fatty acid composition in membranes of cells involved in the immune inflammatory response • Omega-3 fatty acids contain eicosapentaenoic acid and docosahexanoic acid • Block production of proinflammatory mediators through competitive inhibition • Play a role in inflammatory resolution and cellular repair	• Continuous administered enteral omega-3 fatty acids in patients with acute lung injury and acute respiratory distress syndrome is associated with decreased number of ventilator days, ICU length of stay, and incidence of new organ failure • Bolus supplementation of omega-3 fatty acids did show benefit to critically ill medical patients
Glutamine Cellular protection	• Glutamine stores are depleted during stress due to excessive utilization • Glutamine supports barrier and immune function • Glutamine enhances heat shock proteins, which provide stress tolerance and protection from tissue injury and death	• Glutamine supplemented PN is associated with reduced mortality, infection, and hospital length of stay • Parenteral glutamine is not readily available in the United States, has limited stability, and poses an infection concern • Canadian guidelines recommend against combined parenteral and enteral glutamine supplementation, NOT be used in critically ill patients with shock and multiorgan failure, as it was associated with increased mortality based on one level-1 trial
Antioxidants Cellular protection	• Antioxidants can be used by the cell to balance increased levels of cell-damaging reactive oxygen species during critical illness	• Vitamin C, vitamin E, and trace element selenium have been shown to improve patient outcomes in burns, trauma, and mechanically ventilated critically ill patients[13]

Abbreviations: ALI, acute lung injury; ARDS, acute respiratory distress syndrome; ICU, intensive care unit; PN, parenteral nutrition.

Data from Collier BR, Cherry-Bukowiec JR, Mills ME. Trauma, surgery, and burns. In: Mueller CM, editor. The A.S.P.E.N Adult Nutrition Support Core Curriculum. 2nd edition. Silver Spring (MD): American Society for Parenteral and Enteral Nutrition; 2012. p. 392–411.

restarted and carbohydrate introduced, the intracellular cations are redistributed back into the cells for glucose metabolism. This phenomenon is often associated with "refeeding syndrome." When severe, refeeding syndrome can result in respiratory, cardiac, and neuromuscular complications, and can be fatal.[9,50,51] It is important for nurses to be aware of this complication and be able to identify patients at risk.[9,50]

Nutrition is to be initiated cautiously in patients identified as at risk for refeeding syndrome. Electrolyte abnormalities should be corrected before initiation of nutrition and feedings should begin at 25% of caloric goal with 100% of protein needs if possible.[50] Daily laboratory values are necessary to guide electrolyte replacement therapy and advancement of calories to goal. Calories should be advanced only on days that electrolytes are within normal limits. An increase in calories by 25% of goal is a safe approach to advancing nutrients. Goals may take as long as a week to achieve.[50,51]

Stress associated hyperglycemia is a common metabolic complication in critically ill patients. Hyperglycemia has been associated with increased infectious morbidity and mortality in the ICU.[25,48,52] For most adult ICU patients, SCCM guidelines recommend initiation of insulin therapy for blood glucose (BG) higher than 150 mg/dL and to maintain BG absolutely lower than 180 mg/dL and avoid hypoglycemia (BG <70).[52] Some patient populations call for tighter glucose control or higher glycemic thresholds, which is outside of the scope of this discussion. The reader is directed to the "Guidelines for the use of an insulin infusion for the management of hyperglycemia in critically ill patients."[25,48,51,52]

BG monitoring every 6 hours should be performed empirically with initiation of nutrition therapy. Some patients may be especially sensitive to the carbohydrate load and require additional lipids in PN to offset the dextrose calories and decrease insulin requirements. Some specialized enteral formulas with a decreased carbohydrate load have been shown to reduce insulin requirements. When increasing fat in the PN or using reduced carbohydrate enteral formulas, monitoring serum triglycerides is warranted.

Hypertriglyceridemia is associated with overfeeding dextrose calories in PN and infusions of IVFE. Hyperlipidemia can impair the immune response and cause pancreatitis when serum levels become excessive. When administering PN and evaluating tolerance to IVFE, the sedation medication propofol should be taken into account, as it is a 10% IVFE and should be considered a caloric source in all patients in the ICU. Serum triglyceride should be measured on initiation of PN and monitored on a weekly basis. IVFE should be withheld for serum triglyceride higher than 400 mg/mL. Essential fatty acid deficiency can develop within 3 weeks when IVFEs are withheld.[25]

Fatty liver (also known as steatosis) is associated with PN and presents with increased liver enzymes usually within the first 2 weeks of therapy.[25,46] An approach to this side effect is to "cycle" the total PN over 12 to 18 hours, allowing an interruption of nutrient delivery and time for the liver to "rest." PN-associated fatty liver usually resolves on its own and is considered benign.[25,46]

NURSING CONSIDERATIONS

Nursing's role is to advocate for the patient to attain nutritional support therapy. Nurses need to understand the importance of nutrition and the guidelines to ensure that their patients are started on and are receiving appropriate and adequate nutrition support. EN via the gastric route requires a tube placed from the nares or oral cavity to the stomach. This can be easily accomplished with a Salem sump tube or a small-bore feeding tube. Typically an abdominal radiograph is used to confirm gastric placement.

If feeding tube placement is needed in the small bowel, there are more specialized tubes and placement techniques that can be used to achieve this. There are many tube placement techniques to achieve small bowel feeding tube placement that have been identified in the literature. A comprehensive review of these techniques is beyond the scope of this article. All techniques have varying degrees of success, as well as possible adverse problems, associated with them. Blind placement can be used, but is successful only 25% of the time.[53] Other tubes and techniques range from magnet, electromagnetic placement device, use of promotility agents, peristaltic tubes, and use of fluoroscopy or endoscopy. The ideal placement technique would be easily achieved at the bedside to avoid patient transport, have a high success rate and no adverse complications, be easy to train personnel, and be cost-effective. Additionally, if the technique could eliminate or minimize radiographic verification, this would also decrease potential adverse events for the patient.

After tube placement and confirmation of appropriate location, the tube should be marked at the insertion site with a black permanent marker and/or documented in the chart. This allows the nurse to easily assess if the tube is in the correct location or if it has become dislodged in the course of care.

Nurses play a role in screening for malnutrition and can quickly identify those patients at risk. One mechanism that has been proven to work with patients in the ICU is the implementation of a nutrition support algorithm. Oftentimes, nutrition may be overlooked when focusing on other aspects of care, but a protocolized approach to delivering nutrition either by nurses or a dietician has been shown to facilitate early and appropriate nutrition and improved outcomes.[54] A recent study demonstrated improved provision of calories and protein delivery with the implementation of a nutrition support algorithm.[55] The investigators also suggest that there could be further improvements with routine nutrition assessments by a dietitian or nutrition support team.[55]

Monitoring Tolerance of Enteral Feedings and Gastric Residual Volumes

Inadequate enteral feeding can be caused by mechanical problems (occlusions, tube replacements), procedural interruptions, and GI complications (high GRV, vomiting, diarrhea, constipation, abdominal pain, distention, small bowel obstruction).[41] Diarrhea is a common finding in patients receiving EN. Feedings need not be discontinued when diarrhea occurs, as this is often not a result of the EN. Diarrhea is often the result of medications containing sorbitol, other treatments, infectious causes, or altered GI anatomy.[56]

One study found that in medical and coronary care ICU, patient's enteral delivery was reported to achieve only 52% of target goals for these reasons.[17] One reason patients do not received target goals is that ventilated patients in the ICU experience feeding interruptions for 5 to 6 hours daily.[17] Failure to deliver adequate feeding, especially in malnourished patients, has raised concerns about cumulative energy deficit in the first week of admission to the ICU, which then correlates to significantly longer ICU stays, more days on the ventilator, and more infections complications.[31]

Nurses need to assess for tolerance of tube feedings as they are infusing. When gastric feedings are infusing, residuals should be checked every 4 hours. As previously discussed, guidelines suggest that you do not need to stop feedings unless GRV is greater than 500 mL.[13] Abdominal assessment of the patient should also include any complaints of pain, nausea, or vomiting and presence of distention. For patients who have continued increased gastric residuals, it is then warranted to try promotility agents or change to small bowel placement of feeding tubes.[13]

Flushing Feeding Tubes

One problem that frequently occurs with feeding tubes is clogging of the tube. The best way to treat this is to prevent it from occurring in the first place. Tubes should be flushed with 30 mL of warm water every 4 hours, and before or after medications are infused. Always ensure that medications given are fully dissolved or given in the elixir form, also ensure that medications are compatible, as this is often a cause for clogs in the tube. Protein supplements that are given must always be well diluted before injecting into the tube and then flushed thoroughly afterward. Some feeding systems allow for water to be given concomitantly with feedings and this also is a benefit to preventing tube clogs. If a clog does occur, the best method for treating is commercial products. Traditional practices of using carbonated sodas are not indicated and should not be practiced.

To ensure that the patient receives the required caloric intake, the nurse must minimize periods in which enteral feedings are turned off for patient positioning and procedures. The traditional practice of turning feedings off when placing the head of the bed flat for a few minutes to reposition is not based on evidence. Common sense dictates that turning feedings off for a few minutes avoids only a few milliliters of EN; if patients are being fed postpyloric, this practice is all the more not necessary. The problem with this practice is that feedings may be turned off and then forgotten to be restarted. The other practice is to turn feedings off for surgery and procedures, the standard practice of NPO at midnight is a tradition-based practice that is not based on evidence and often results in decreased caloric intake and inability to reach the goal of feedings. This is especially true with postpyloric feedings. Anesthesia guidelines recommend preoperative fasting of solids up to 6 hours and clear fluids 2 hours preoperatively.[56,57] Other research studies also support that there is feasibility and safety (no increase in adverse events) in continuing enteral feedings up to and sometimes during the operative period, when feedings are delivered postpyloric in the small bowel.[58–60] The research is limited, includes small sample sizes, and would benefit from larger randomized trials.

SUMMARY

Malnutrition is a major concern for critically ill patients and has significant consequences if not identified and treated proactively. The best course of action would be prevention of malnutrition in these patients, but often the patient has already had decreased nutritional intake before entering the hospital. Nutrition risk assessment is essential to identify patients who are malnourished or are at increased risk for developing malnutrition and to prevent further loss of lean body mass and improve patient outcomes.

The safe provision of nutrition is essential in patients in the ICU and includes ongoing assessment of risk and early EN. The ICU nurse should be knowledgeable of clinically applicable protocols and techniques to facilitate early EN in this vulnerable patient population. Nurses also need to be cognizant of potential adverse consequences associated with nutritional therapies and be proactive in preventing and early recognition of complications if they occur. The ICU nurse is in the best position to advocate for appropriate nutritional therapies and to facilitate the safe delivery of nutrition.

REFERENCES

1. Jensen GL, Mirtallo J, Copher C, et al. Adult starvation and disease-related malnutrition: a proposal for etiology-based diagnosis in the clinical practice

setting from the International Consensus Guideline Committee. Clin Nutr 2010; 291:151–3.

2. Wischmeyer PE. Malnutrition in the acutely ill patient: is it more than just protein and energy? S Afr J Clin Nutr 2011;24(3). S1-S7.

3. Middleton MH, Nazerenko G, Nivison-Smith I, et al. Prevalence of malnutrition and 12-month incidence of mortality in two Sydney teaching hospitals. Intern Med J 2001;31:455–61.

4. Bauer JD, Isenring E, Torma J, et al. Nutritional status of patients who have fallen in an acute care setting. J Hum Nutr Diet 2007;20:558–64.

5. Vivanti A, Ward N, Haines T. Nutritional status and associations with falls, balance, mobility and functionality during hospital admission. J Nutr Health Aging 2011;15(5):388–91.

6. Somanchi M, Tao X, Mullin GE. The facilitated early enteral and dietary management effectiveness trial in hospitalized patients with malnutrition. JPEN J Parenter Enteral Nutr 2011;35(2):209–16.

7. Codner PA. Enteral nutrition in the critically ill patient. Surg Clin North Am 2012; 92:1485–501.

8. Wischmeyer P. Nutritional pharmacology in surgery and critical care: you must unlearn what you have learned. Cur Opin Anesth 2011;24:381–6.

9. Hiesmayr M. Nutrition risk assessment in the ICU. Curr Opin Clin Nutr Metab Care 2012;15(2):174–80.

10. White JV, Guenter P, Jensen G, et al, The Academy Malnutrition Work Group, the A.S.P.E.N. Manutrition Task Force, A.S.P.E.N. Board of Directors. Consensus statement: Academy of Nutrition and Dietetics and American Society for Parenteral and Enteral Nutrition: Characteristics Recommended for the Identification and Documentation of Adult Malnutrition (Undernutrition). JPEN J Parenter Enteral Nutr 2012;36(3):275–83.

11. Jensen GL. Inflammation as the key interface of the medical and nutrition universes: a provocative examination of the future of clinical nutrition and medicine. JPEN J Parenter Enteral Nutr 2006;30:453–63.

12. Wagenmakers AJ. Muscle function in critically ill patients. Clin Nutr 2001;20(5): 451–4.

13. McClave SA, Martindale BG, Vanek VW, et al, A.S.P.E.N. Board of Directors, American College of Critical Care Medicine. Guidelines for the Provision and Assessment of Nutrition Support Therapy in the Adult Critically Ill Patient: Society of Critical Care Medicine (SCCM) and American Society for Parenteral and Enteral Nutrition. JPEN J Parenter Enteral Nutr 2009;33:277–316.

14. Collier BR, Cherry-Bukowiec JR, Mills ME. Trauma, surgery, and burns. In: Mueller CM, editor. The A.S.P.E.N Adult Nutrition Support Core Curriculum. 2nd edition. Silver Spring (MD): American Society for Parenteral and Enteral Nutrition; 2012. p. 392–411.

15. Heyland DK, Dhaliwal R, Drover JW, et al. Canadian clinical practice guidelines for nutrition support in mechanically ventilated, critically ill adult patients. JPEN J Parenter Enteral Nutr 2003;27:355–73.

16. Artinian V, Krayem H, DiGiovine B. Effects of early enteral feeding on the outcome of critically ill mechanically ventilated medical patients. Chest 2006; 129:960–7.

17. McClave SA, Sexton LK, Spain DA, et al. Enteral tube feeding in the intensive care unit: factors impeding adequate delivery. Crit Care Med 1999;27:1252–6.

18. Dickerson RN. Optimal caloric intake for critically ill patients: first, do no harm. Nutr Clin Pract 2011;26:48–54.

19. Berger MM, Chiolero RL, Pannatier A, et al. A 10-year survey of nutritional support in a surgical ICU: 1986-1995. Nutrition 1997;13:870–7.
20. Mueller C, Compher C, Druyan ME. Nutrition screening, assessment, and intervention in adults. JPEN J Parenter Enteral Nutr 2011;35(1):16–24.
21. Alberda C, Gramlich L, Jones N, et al. The relationship between nutritional intake and clinical outcomes in critically ill patients: results of an international multicenter observational study. Intensive Care Med 2009;35:1728–37.
22. Berger MM, Pichard C. Best timing for energy provision during critical illness. Crit Care 2012;16:215–22.
23. Cerrra FB, Benitez MR, Blackburn GL, et al. Applied nutrition in ICU patients: a consensus statement of the American College of Chest Physicians. Chest 1997; 111:769–78.
24. Talpers SS, Romberger DJ, Bunce SB, et al. Nutritionally associated increased carbon dioxide production. Excess total calories vs. high proportion of carbohydrate calories. Chest 1992;102:551–5.
25. Reid C. Frequency of under- and overfeeding in mechanically ventilated ICU patients: causes and possible consequences. Hum Nutr Dietet 2006;19:13–22.
26. Kaminski DL, Adams A, Jellinek M. The effect of hyperalimentation on hepatic lipid content and lipogenic enzyme activity in rats and man. Surgery 1980;88: 93–100.
27. Kumpf VJ, Gervasio JG. Complications of parenteral nutrition. In: Mueller CM, editor. The ASPEN Adult Nutrition Support Curriculum. Silver Spring (MD): American Society for Parenteral and Enteral Nutrition; 2012. p. 284–97.
28. Skipper A, Tupesis N. Is there a role for nonprotein calories in developing and evaluating the nutrition prescription? Nutr Clin Pract 2005;20:321–4.
29. Cherry-Bukowiec JR. Optimizing nutrition therapy to enhance mobility in critically ill patients. Crit Care Nurs Q 2013;36(1):28–36.
30. Krishnan KA, Parce PB, Martinez A, et al. Caloric intake in medical ICU patients. Chest 2003;124:297–305.
31. Villet S, Chiolero RL, Bollmann MD, et al. Negative impact of hypocaloric feeding and energy balance on clinical outcome in ICU patients. Clin Nutr 2005;24: 502–9.
32. Cassaer MP, Mesotten D, Hermans G, et al. Early versus late parenteral nutrition in critically ill adults. N Engl J Med 2011;365:506–17.
33. Heidegger CP, Berger MM, Graf S, et al. Optimization of energy provision with supplemental parenteral nutrition in critically ill patients: a randomized controlled clinical trial. Lancet 2013;381:385–93.
34. Singer P, Anbar R, Cohen J, et al. The tight calorie control study (TICACOS): a prospective, randomized, controlled pilot study of nutritional support critically ill patients. Intensive Care Med 2011;37:601–9.
35. Kondrup J. Can food intake in hospitals be improved? Clin Nutr 2001;20: 153–60.
36. De Jonghe B, Appere-De-Vechi C, Fournier M, et al. A prospective survey of nutritional support practices in intensive care unit patients? What is prescribed? What is delivered? Crit Care Med 2001;29:8–12.
37. Heyland DK, Schroter-Noppe D, Drover JW, et al. Nutrition support in the critical care setting: current practice in Canadian ICUs—opportunities for improvement? JPEN J Parenter Enteral Nutr 2003;27:74–83.
38. Heimburger DC. Adulthood in modern nutrition. In: Shike M, Ross AC, Cabellero B, et al, editors. Health and disease, vol. 53. New York: Lippincott Williams & Wilkins; 2006. p. 830–42.

39. Rice TW, Swope T, Bozeman S, et al. Variation in enteral nutrition delivery in mechanically ventilated patients. Nutrition 2005;21:786–92.

40. Btaiche IF, Lingtak-Neander C, Pleva M, et al. Critical illness, gastrointestinal complications, and medications therapy during enteral feeding in critically ill adult patients. Nutr Clin Pract 2010;25:32–49.

41. Heyland DK, Wishmeyer PE. The future of critical care nutrition therapy. Crit Care Clin 2010;26:433–41.

42. Ukleja A. Altered GI motility in critically ill patients: current understanding of pathophysiology, clinical impact, and diagnostic approach. Nutr Clin Pract 2010;25:16–25.

43. Chapman JM, Nguyen NQ, Fraser JL. Current and future therapeutic prokinetic therapy to improve enteral feed intolerance in the ICU patient. Nutr Clin Pract 2010;25:26–31.

44. Elamin EM, Camporesi E. Evidence-based nutritional support in the intensive care unit. Int Anesthesiol Clin 2009;47(1):121–38.

45. Zhongheng Zhang MM, Xiao Xu MB, Jin Ding HN. Comparison of postpyloric tube feeding and gastric tube feeding in intensive care unit patients: a meta-analysis. Nutr Clin Pract 2013;28(3):371–80.

46. Ziegler TR. Parenteral nutrition in the critically ill patient. N Engl J Med 2009;361:1088–97.

47. O'Grady NP, Alexander M, Burns LA, et al. Guidelines for the prevention of intravascular catheter related infection. 2011. Available at: http://www.cdc.gov/HAI/bsi/bsi.html. Accessed September 16, 2013.

48. Mirtallo JM, Patel M. Overview of parenteral nutrition. In: Mueller CM, editor. The A.S.P.E.N. Adult Nutrition Support Core Curriculum. Silver Spring (MD): American Society for Parenteral and Enteral Nutrition; 2012. p. 234–44.

49. Task Force for the Revision of Safe Practices for Parenteral Nutrition, Canada T, Johnson D, Kumpf V, et al. Safe practices for parenteral nutrition. JPEN J Parenter Enteral Nutr 2004;28:S39–70.

50. Kraft MD, Btaiche IF, Sacks GS. Review of the refeeding syndrome. Nutr Clin Pract 2005;20:625–33.

51. Adkins SM. Recognizing and preventing refeeding syndrome. Dimens Crit Care Nurs 2009;29(2):53–8.

52. Jacobi J, Bircher N, Krinsley J, et al. Guidelines for the use of an insulin infusion for the management of hyperglycemia in critically ill patients. Crit Care Med 2012;40:3251–76.

53. Hernandez-Socorro CR, Marin J, Ruiz-Santana S, et al. Bedside sonographic-guided versus blind nasoenteric feeding tube placement in critically ill patients. Crit Care Med 1996;24(10):1690–4.

54. Soguel L, Revelly JP, Schaller MD, et al. Energy deficit and length of hospital stay can be reduced by a two-step quality improvement of nutrition therapy: the intensive care unit dietitian can make the difference. Crit Care Med 2012;40(2):412–9.

55. Kiss CM, Byham-Gray L, Denmark R, et al. The impact of a implementation of a nutrition support algorithm on nutrition care outcomes in an intensive care unit. Nutr Clin Pract 2012;23(6):793–801.

56. Parrish CR, McCray S. Enteral feeding: dispelling myths. Pract Gastroenterol 2003;9:33–50.

57. Smith AF. Preoperative fasting in adults. In: Colvin JR, Peden CJ, editors. Raising the standard: a compendium of audit recipes: section 1, preoperative care. London: Royal College of Anaesthetists; 2012. p. 67. Available at: http://www.rcoa.ac.uk/system/files/CSQ-ARB-2012.pdf. Accessed August 30, 2013.

58. Pousman RM, Pepper C, Pandharipande P, et al. Feasibility of implementing a reduced fasting protocol for critically ill trauma patients undergoing operative and nonoperative procedures. JPEN J Parenter Enteral Nutr 2009;33(2):176–80.
59. McElroy LM, Codner PA, Brasel KJ. A pilot study to explore the safety of perioperative postpyloric enteral nutrition. Nutr Clin Pract 2012;27:777–80.
60. Moncure M, Samaha E, Moncure K, et al. Jejunostomy tube feedings should not be stopped in the perioperative patient. JPEN J Parenter Enteral Nutr 1999; 23(6):356–9.

Nutrition and Care Considerations in the Overweight and Obese Population Within the Critical Care Setting

Jody Collins, MSN, RN

KEYWORDS

- Obesity • Overweight • Bariatric • Body mass index • Critical illness • Nutrition

KEY POINTS

- Care and nutritional support for obese critically ill patients is complex.
- Unique care considerations and complications for overweight and obese critically ill patients exist and must be understood to provide optimal support during hospitalization.

INTRODUCTION

Growing concern among health care providers exists regarding the continued projected increase in worldwide obesity. The prevalence of overweight and obesity has increased steadily among all groups of Americans over the past 3 decades.[1] Key findings related to obesity in the 2009–2010 Health and Nutrition Examination Survey revealed that more than one-third of adults and approximately 17% of youth in America were obese.[2] That compromises 35.7% of the population and is one of the leading health issues in US society, resulting in about 300,000 deaths per year in the United States. Today, about 65% of Americans are now considered either overweight or obese.[2] Nearly one-third of patients in the critical care setting meet the criteria for obesity, and up to 7% are morbidly obese.[3] Patients with obesity present management challenges when they are in the critical care setting, from both the comorbidities that accompany their illness and the differences in management that they require.[3]

OBESITY DEFINED

Excess weight and obesity were not always viewed as a health risk. Historically, being overweight or obese was seen as a sign of elite eminence and wealth. In contrast,

Conflict of Interest/Financial Disclosure Statement: The author declares no conflict of interest or financial interests to disclose relating to the content of this article.
Clinical Projects and Magnet Program, Memorial Hermann The Woodlands Hospital, 9250 Pinecroft, The Woodlands, TX 77380, USA
E-mail address: Jodyc42@gmail.com

during times of struggle and historical turmoil, food was seen as a scarce commodity, a vital necessity for substance of life and endurance for daily function.[4] Today, more often than not, historical perspective conflicts with individual class or station identification regarding weight status. In fact, as our state of living continues to evolve, we are seeing greater increases in individual body mass and size, threatening the overall health and well-being on a global perspective.[5]

Obesity is the fastest-growing chronic condition in the United States, affecting greater than 30% of the adult population. Obesity is defined as having a very high amount of body fat in relation to lean body mass or body mass index (BMI) of 30 or greater. Overweight and obesity are both labels for ranges of weight that are greater than what is generally considered healthy for a given height. Both considered a significant risk to health status, they are defined as abnormal or excessive fat accumulation. Weight status is typically measured by BMI, a person's weight (in kilograms) divided by the square of his or her height (in centimeters). A person with a BMI equal to or more than 25 is considered overweight, whereas a BMI of 30 or more is generally considered obese.[4] Specific labels and BMI ranges have been updated and include definitions for obesity from the World Health Organization (**Table 1**).[5]

For optimum health, the median BMI for an adult population should be in the range of 21 to 23 kg/m^2, whereas the goal for individuals should be to maintain BMI in the range 18.5 to 24.9 kg/m^2.[6] Weight loss is recommended for individuals who are considered obese (BMI greater than or equal to 30) or those who are identified as overweight (BMI of 25.0–29.9) and have 2 or more contributing risk factors. An overall weight loss (between 5% and 10% of actual weight) can lower the individual risk of developing diseases associated with obesity. Prevention of further weight gain, rather than weight loss, may prevent overweight individuals from developing contributing risk factors. Individuals should consult with a health care practitioner to evaluate the risk factors and BMI for increased risk.[7]

OBESITY PREVALENCE

The World Health Organization (WHO) projected an increase in the number of obese individuals to 700 million by the year 2015.[5] In a 2008 WHO study, 35% of adults aged 20 years and older were overweight (BMI ≥ 25 kg/m^2), 34% of men and 35% of women. Worldwide prevalence of obesity has nearly doubled between the years of 1980 and 2008. The WHO study also revealed 10% of men and 14% of women in the world were obese (BMI ≥ 30 kg/m^2) compared with 5% for men and 8% for women in 1980. An estimated 205 million men and 297 million women older than 20 years were considered to be obese, estimating more than half a billion adults worldwide.[5]

Table 1 Obesity classifications	
Overweight	25.0–29.9 kg/m^2
Class I obesity (moderate)	30.0–34.9 kg/m^2
Class II obesity (severe)	35.0–39.9 kg/m^2
Class III obesity (commonly called severe or morbid obesity)	>40 kg/m^2 BMI: 40.0–49.9 kg/m^2 morbidly obese BMI: >50 kg/m^2 super obese

Data from World Health Organization. Obesity and overweight fact sheet. 2013. Available at: http://www.who.int/mediacentre/factsheets/fs311/en/index.html. Accessed August 12, 2013.

Over the past 10 to 15 years, there has been a dramatic increase in obesity across the United States. In a state-by-state comparison, no state met the nation's Healthy People 2010 goal to reduce the prevalence of obesity to 15%. In 2010, there were 12 states with an obesity prevalence of 30%. The US history of obesity prevalence is shown in **Table 2**.[2]

Although it varies depending on the comparison group, prevalence estimates among critically ill patients may be as high as 1 in 4 patients. For obesity, the difference more than triples from 7% obesity in both sexes in lower-middle-income countries to 24% in upper-middle-income countries. Women's obesity was significantly higher than men's, with the exception of high-income countries where it was similar. In low- and lower-middle-income countries, obesity among women was approximately double that among men.[5] For the age group of 40 to 59 year olds, the obesity prevalence is more than 40%.[8] Minority women are disproportionately affected, with greater than 50% of non-Hispanic black women and Mexican American women aged 40 to 59 years being obese.[9]

Obesity increases the risk of many health conditions, and intensive care unit (ICU) providers should be aware of the possible physiologic changes occurring with obesity that may become relevant during critical illness. Obesity complicates care during critical illness, including challenging physiologic changes occurring with corpulence. Special challenges that are encountered when caring for obese patients in the critical care setting include airway management, nutritional support, drug dosing, bedside procedures, testing, and overall nursing care.[10]

CARE CONSIDERATIONS

The obese patient population has an essential set of care requirements; when health care professionals are knowledgeable in these requirements, the overall care is more than likely to benefit the patient population and provide a more positive healing environment. The care considerations of critically ill obese patients can involve difficulties with mobilization and positioning, size-appropriate furnishings, and supplies and instruments; the absence of appropriate monitoring and diagnostic equipment for hemodynamic monitoring and irregularity of pharmacokinetic effects put these patients at an increased risk for skin breakdown and wound healing.[11] Contributing factors that heighten risks include overweight and obese patients having greater abdominal fat deposits, which is linked with insulin resistance, hyperglycemia, and an increased risk of death.[12] Abdominal adiposity of obesity is strongly associated with metabolic syndrome.[13] The National Cholesterol Education Program's Adult Treatment Panel III report from 2002 defined metabolic syndrome as a clustering of risk factors with primary clinical outcomes of cardiovascular disease and insulin resistance,[14] thus increasing complications and may warrant hospitalization.[15]

Critical care providers need to have a heightened awareness of the variable physiologic changes that may occur with overweight and obese patients during critical illness. Some conditions within this patient population associated with and needing special attention include the physiologic consequences of obesity: cardiovascular, respiratory, and renal complications.

From a cardiac standpoint, overweight and obese patients are frequently deconditioned and have an increased incidence of coronary artery disease. These patients typically have a higher resting heart rate or resting tachycardia that may degrade during the progression of critical illness.[3] Obesity can cause significant alterations in overall cardiac performance and structure and is characterized by an increase in total blood volume and resting cardiac output. The increase in cardiac output is related

Table 2
US history of obesity prevalence

	2010 US Obesity Rates						
State	US Obese Adults (%) (BMI ≥30)	State	US Obese Adults (%) (BMI ≥30)	State	US Obese Adults (%) (BMI ≥30)	State	US Obese Adults (%) (BMI ≥30)
Alabama	32.2	Illinois	28.2	Montana	23.0	Rhode Island	25.5
Alaska	24.5	Indiana	29.6	Nebraska	26.9	South Carolina	31.5
Arizona	24.3	Iowa	28.4	Nevada	22.4	South Dakota	27.3
Arkansas	30.1	Kansas	29.4	New Hampshire	25.0	Tennessee	30.8
California	24.0	Kentucky	31.3	New Jersey	23.8	Texas	31.0
Colorado	21.0	Louisiana	31.0	New Mexico	25.1	Utah	22.5
Connecticut	22.5	Maine	26.8	New York	23.9	Vermont	23.2
Delaware	28.0	Maryland	27.1	North Carolina	27.8	Virginia	26.0
District of Columbia	22.2	Massachusetts	23.0	North Dakota	27.2	Washington	25.5
Florida	26.6	Michigan	30.9	Ohio	29.2	West Virginia	32.5
Georgia	29.6	Minnesota	24.8	Oklahoma	30.4	Wisconsin	26.3
Hawaii	22.7	Mississippi	34.0	Oregon	26.8	Wyoming	25.1
Idaho	26.5	Missouri	30.5	Pennsylvania	28.6	—	

Adapted from Centers for Disease Control and Prevention, Division of Nutrition, Physical Activity, and Obesity. The history of state obesity prevalence (from 1985–2010). Available at: http://www.cdc.gov/obesity/data/adult.html#History. Accessed August 16, 2013.

solely to an increase in stroke volume, with the heart rate being unchanged.[16] Blood volume and effect on preload increases as body mass and stroke volume increases, thus augmenting cardiac output as a compensatory response to the increased metabolic demands caused by the excess body weight. Therefore, the resting cardiac output,[16] preload, and tension of the cardiac wall increase, all potentially leading the left ventricle to develop eccentric hypertrophy.[16] Obese patients with a BMI greater than 40 kg/m² and those with a long duration of substantial obesity are especially vulnerable to cardiovascular compromise.[17] It is not surprising that obese critically ill patients may not tolerate large volume shifts and aggressive fluid resuscitation. Care management for this patient population is additionally complicated by body habitus, with challenges during physical examination in assessing volume status; assessment using echocardiography is also hampered by technical limitations in obese patients.[17]

The effect of obesity on lung function is complex and is influenced by the degree of obesity, age, and type of body fat distribution. The physiologic changes and management of the respiratory system should be anticipated in obese patients.[17] Overweight and obese patients are at an increased risk of developing respiratory complications,[18] which may be in the form of increased incidence of conditions such as asthma or sleep apnea. Young and colleagues[19] demonstrated a significant sleep apnea prevalence of approximately 40% in moderately overweight men who are otherwise healthy[20]; there is between 40% and 90% prevalence in severely obese men with a BMI greater than 40 kg/m².[18,21–27]

Patients who are morbidly obese and have obstructive sleep apnea (OSA) have an increased incidence of cor pulmonale and pulmonary hypertension that may make the monitoring of central venous pressures less reliable, but rarely will OSA interfere with other management unless it is a known diagnosis before the illness.[17] Health care providers can have greater difficulties managing the airway of patients in pulmonary failure or experience challenges with ventilation and weaning patients who are morbidly obese.[3] Patients with severe obesity usually present with a widened alveolar-arterial oxygen gradient caused by ventilation-perfusion mismatching, therefore, causing hypoxemia.[28] Alveolar collapse and airway closure at the bases contribute to this occurrence. When in the supine position, the functional residual capacity (FRC) decreases, further increasing ventilation-perfusion challenges, resulting in severe arterial hypoxemia and sudden death.[29] Anesthesia further reduces the FRC, with the impingement of the FRC on the closing volume.[11] When FRC is sufficiently reduced, it can approach the closing capacity and lead to small airway closure. Along with the increases in blood volume seen in the pulmonary circulation, this contributes to decreased lung compliance.[30]

Anatomic changes also occur in the airways. Upper airway caliber decreases because of parapharyngeal fat deposition. Airways tend to be more collapsible for a variety of reasons, but important factors include impaired pharyngeal dilator activity because of altered pharyngeal shape. Airway caliber may also be affected by remodeling that occurs in response to inflammatory adipocytokines or from repeated opening and closing of the airways during tidal breathing that leads to atelectrauma.[10] Ultimately, higher airway resistance increases the work of breathing. Because of the constant increased load on the respiratory muscles, the oxygen cost of breathing is substantially higher for obese patients.[31] As oxygen consumption by the respiratory muscles increases, endurance decreases, as measured by maximum voluntary ventilation maneuvers (20% reduction in patients with simple obesity and 45% reduction in patients with morbid obesity).[32] In sum, obese individuals, particularly the morbidly obese, have significantly reduced respiratory reserve to compensate for critical illness.

The changes in pulmonary function of obese patients have significant effects on assisted mechanical ventilation and predominantly in ventilator management. Because the lung volumes can be reduced and airway resistance increased, tidal volume calculated according to patients' actual body weight is likely to lead to high overall airway pressures and alveolar overdistension. The initial tidal volume should be based on the ideal body weight (IBW) and adjusted according to blood gas concentrations and inflation pressures. Inflation pressures should be interpreted with caution because compliance of the total respiratory system (both lung and chest wall) is reduced and airway resistance is increased in obese patients when compared with normal subjects.[33] This set of circumstances results in higher peak and static airway pressures than are generally recommended and may be required for adequate alveolar ventilation without causing alveolar overdistension in obese patients.[33] Therefore, the use of positive end-expiratory pressure is recommended as it may prevent end-expiratory airway closure and atelectasis, particularly in dorsal lung regions.[33] Because of the increased risk of aspiration, reduced pulmonary defense mechanisms, and basal atelectasis, mechanically ventilated obese patients are at an increased risk of developing ventilator-associated pneumonia.

The prevalence of acute kidney injury during critical illness among obese patients is unknown. Between the propensities toward diabetic nephropathy and hypertensive renal disease, patients with morbid obesity can show very little renal reserve and decreases in renal function.[5] Glomerular filtration rate evaluation is challenging in this patient population because the estimating formulas used have limitations when used during critical illness because of the dynamic fluid, metabolic, hemodynamic, and hormonal changes.[3] Obese individuals may have glomerular hyperfiltration[34] and higher creatinine generation caused by increases in both fat and lean body mass as total body weight increases. Weight-based creatinine clearance estimating formulas have been developed to accommodate obese patients, but further investigation is needed to endorse these formulas.[10] Timed or 24-hour urine collections can provide more accurate estimations of renal function in the critical care setting but may not always be practical.[10] Adding to this complexity, obese patients often have multiple comorbidities that predispose them to chronic kidney disease.[10] Kidney dysfunction can develop for a variety of reasons, including iatrogenic prerenal azotemia resulting from overly aggressive diuresis, particularly when a challenging physical examination is combined with a history of cardiac disease; complaints of dyspnea; and findings of peripheral edema. In addition, medications for weight loss or previous bariatric surgery may lead to fat malabsorption, which can make obese patients prone to the development of acute oxalate nephropathy.[33]

Health care providers need to be aware that management and the necessary supportive care, such as renal replacement therapy, requiring vascular access may be challenging because of the difficulties in obtaining vascular access for initiation for dialysis. Compounding this challenge is the fact that the methods to precisely calculate the dialysis dose, such as continuous venovenous hemofiltration (CVVH), are not well established in this patient population. A study by Ronco and colleagues[35] showed that weight-based CVVH dosing of at least 35 mL/kg/min improved survival when compared with a lower dose of 20 mL/kg/min in a general ICU population; however, the average weight of patients in this cohort was around 70 kg, with a standard deviation of approximately 10 kg. Among morbidly obese patients, dosing based on actual weight leads to an impractical, large, and possibly unsafe volume of replacement fluid. Although there is a lack of evidence, estimated lean body weight adjustments should probably be used for dose calculations.[28]

Critical care obese patients are at a higher risk of systemic inflammatory response syndrome leading to multiple organ dysfunction syndrome (MODS).[6,36–38] Conditions of hypotension, hypoxia, and hypoperfusion are considered end points of MODS that decrease overall tissue perfusion and increase a patient's risk of skin breakdown. Factors that influence skin breakdown, such as sedation, use of paralytics, fluid overload, fever, incontinence, and mechanical trauma, are particularly important to assess in obese critical care patients.[33] Overweight and obese patients are at a staggering risk for the development of pressure ulcers for several reasons. The decreased perfusion of adipose tissue puts that tissue and the overlying skin at risk for reduced blood flow. The excessive weight load of the patients and the body part in contact with the mattress, combined with localized low blood flow, makes these patients susceptible to the development of pressure ulcers up to weeks after an episode of shock. Limitations caused by the patients' size and weight include difficulty turning and maintaining in a turned position; thus, patients who are expected to be in bed for more than a few days should have a special bed or mattress, preferably one that has low air-loss surfaces with options for pressure relief.[5] Early recognition and treatment of pressure ulcers is necessary and includes daily inspection and frequent scheduled turning. Approximately one-third of ICU patients are obese, making these patients more likely to have increased lengths of stay, higher morbidity, and increased likelihood of discharge to nursing home facilities.[11,29,30,39] Procurement of specialized bariatric equipment, such as movable sliding air mattresses, patient lifts, and specialized bed chairs, and other special equipment, such as blood pressure cuffs and laryngoscope handles, may be warranted.

The combination of being critically ill and obese present difficult challenges to care, ranging from basic care needs of positioning and mobility to more complicated issues, such as medication management, dosing, and ventilator control. It takes a team of caregivers to coordinate care for overweight and obese patients from lifting considerations to nutrition support. The development of a specialized team of bariatric experts to consult on mobility and care issues for these patients is vital in promoting patient and staff safety and ensuring the best possible dignified care for patients with morbid obesity.

NUTRITIONAL SUPPORT

As expected, with the upward trend of people being larger than in past years, a growing number of critical care patients are overweight or obese. Thirty percent to 35% of adult ICU patients are considered obese and some 5% morbidly obese.[3,38] The risk and demand to adequately provide nutritional support for critical care patients are intensified for health care providers when patients are obese.[3] With the growing levels of overweight and obese patients, metabolic syndrome, and bariatric surgery for weight loss, the prevalence of obesity has increased approximately 10-fold since the late 1960s and doubled since the early 1990s. As of 2002, an estimated 22% of US adults have been identified with metabolic syndrome; an increasing number of Americans, some estimated 220,000, have undergone weight loss procedures since 2008.[28]

At first glance, critically ill obese patients may not seem to present difficulties with nutrition; however, obesity and malnutrition can coexist during critical illness, and providing appropriate nutritional support is essential.[10] In comparison with nonobese patients, obese patients in the ICU typically have challenges effecting responses to stress,[3] such as higher glucose levels with inflated responses to stress; higher insulin levels with lower responses to stress; higher cortisol levels with normal responses to stress; higher norepinephrine and epinephrine levels with decreased response to stress; lower human growth hormone levels but normal response to stress; and higher levels of ketones and free fatty acids and normal resting energy expenditure with higher muscle and nitrogen loss in the ICU.[3]

All patients entering the critical care unit should have a nutritional screen completed within 48 hours of admission. Those patients that are determined to be at risk should have a complete nutritional assessment done by a nutritional expert. Because patients with obesity experience more complications, it is recommended that they have an assessment and nutritional support plan in place within 48 hours of admission.[40]

Excess carbon dioxide production may result from overfeeding, thus, prolong ventilator days in this already vulnerable patient population. Furthermore, overfeeding may intensify hyperglycemia, azotemia, and hepatic fat accumulation.[10] In an effort to minimize issues associated with overfeeding and allowing for a net positive nitrogen balance, the idea of hypocaloric, high-protein feeding has been promoted to facilitate overall fat loss. In 2009, both the Society of Critical Care Medicine and the American Society for Parenteral and Enteral Nutrition endorsed the use of hypocaloric enteral feeding for obese ICU patients, providing no more than 60% to 70% of the target caloric requirements or 11 to 14 kcal/kg actual body weight daily.[3,40] They recommend delivering at least 2.0 g/kg IBW per day as protein in class I and II obesity and at least 2.5 g/kg IBW per day for class III obesity. There are contraindications to this approach for patients with severe renal and hepatic dysfunction whereby a high protein load is detrimental, require a full caloric load, such as with recurring hypoglycemia or severe immunocompromised state.[3,40]

Because of a lack of validated formulas, target caloric intake assessment is difficult. Using indirect calorimetry may provide helpful suggestions but, at times, nonpractical calculations. For example, with the Harris-Benedict equation, there are shortcomings when using IBW as well as actual body weight. Some researchers have advocated the use of an obesity-adjusted weight with a 25% correction of excess weight more than the IBW as follows.[27] The adjusted body weight = (actual weight − IBW) 0.25 + IBW. The recommendations of the "A.S.P.E.N. Clinical Guidelines: Nutrition Support of Hospitalized Adult Patients with Obesity" include that the Pennsylvania State University's 2010 predictive equation or modified version be used to calculate the energy requirements for patients older than 60 years.[40]

Despite excess fat stores, obese patients can rapidly develop protein calorie malnutrition during critical illness. This malnutrition is caused in part by increased baseline insulin levels suppressing lipid mobilization from fat stores and enhancing protein breakdown to fuel gluconeogenesis.[3]

Obese trauma patients have benefitted from a protein-sparing hypocaloric formula and tight glucose control (TGC). A recent randomized study in general adult ICUs demonstrated a significant reduction in mortality for obese patients treated with TGC compared with a conventional glycemic control group (16.7% vs 51.4%, respectively; $P<.01$).[41] Other earlier studies found that insulin secreted in response to continuous infusion of glucose during total parenteral nutrition (TPN) reduced lipolysis as well as the favorable effects of starvation ketosis during trauma-induced negative calorie balance.[42]

It is recommended that TPN be administered in hypocaloric dosages to overweight and obese patients, and it is recommended that these patients receive sufficient nitrogen in order to promote adequate wound healing and combat infection.[42] Protein dosage can be administered in levels of up to 2 g/kg of IBW in these patients and may help preserve lean body mass and reduce adipose tissue.[41] By increasing lean body mass and improving skeletal muscle insulin sensitivity and overall fitness,[43] a preoperative progressive resistance training protocol may ultimately reduce patients' perioperative risk.[28,43]

Patients who have undergone bariatric surgical procedures are at an increased risk for nutrient deficiencies. These deficiencies are caused by the restrictive and malabsorption aspects of the different procedures used for weight loss. Hospitalized patients who have undergone these procedures should be evaluated for deficiencies of iron, copper, selenium, thiamine, zinc, folate, and vitamins D and B12.[40] Replacement of these nutrients should be addressed and taken into consideration for nutritional support. Bariatric procedures also lead to limitations related to placement of feeding tubes. Care must be taken when placing feeding tubes in this patient population so as to not cause injury and may need to be placed endoscopically.

SUMMARY

Patients with morbid obesity present many challenges to their care in the ICU; but with proper management, they can enjoy treatment success near to that of nonobese patients. Multidisciplinary experts, including pharmacists and dietitians, with specialized experience with overweight and obese populations should be part of the overall care plan for these individuals to ensure that adequate and sufficient nutritional support is provided.[3] Further research, including clinically meaningful and quantifiable outcomes, is necessary to fully understand the nutrition support within the critical care setting.

ACKNOWLEDGMENTS

The author expresses her gratitude to Miranda Kelly, DNP, APRN, ACNP-BC for her continual support and diligence and coordination for this project and to Jan Foster, PhD, APRN, CNS, CCRN for her mentorship and support during the preparation of this article.

REFERENCES

1. Ogden CL, Carroll MD, Curtin LR, et al. Prevalence of overweight and obesity in the United States, 1999–2004. JAMA 2006;295(13):1549–55.
2. Centers for Disease Control and Prevention, Division of Nutrition, Physical Activity, and Obesity. Available at: http://www.cdc.gov/obesity/data/adult.html#History. Accessed August 16, 2013.
3. Brusco L. (2011). Critical care of the morbidly obese patient. Current concepts (adult) 14th edition Congress. 2010. Available at: http://www.learnicu.org/Lists/LearningObjectLibrary_object/Attachments/18/Chapter%209.pdf. Accessed August 12, 2013.
4. Ogden CL, Carroll MD, Kit BK, et al. Prevalence of obesity in the United States, 2009–2010. Available at: http://www.cdc.gov/obesity/data/adult.html#Common. Accessed August 12, 2013.
5. World Health Organization. Obesity and overweight fact sheet. 2013. Available at: http://www.who.int/topics/obesity/en/. Accessed August 12, 2013.
6. Oliveros H, Villamor E. Obesity and mortality in critically ill adults: a systematic review and meta-analysis. Obesity (Silver Spring) 2008;16(3):515–21.
7. National Institutes of Health. Available at: http://www.nhlbi.nih.gov/health/public/heart/obesity/lose_wt/bmi_dis.htm. Accessed September 13, 2013.
8. Ogden CL, Yanovski SZ, Carroll MD, et al. The epidemiology of obesity. Gastroenterology 2007;132(6):2087–102.

9. Ogden CL. Disparities in obesity prevalence in the United States: black women at risk. Am J Clin Nutr 2009;89(4):1001–2.
10. Honiden S, McArdle JR. Obesity in the intensive care unit. Clin Chest Med 2009; 30(3):581–99.
11. Bearden DT, Rodvold KA. Dosage adjustments for antibacterials in obese patients: applying clinical pharmacokinetics. Clin Pharm 2000;38(5):415–26.
12. McCowen KC, Malhotra A, Bistrian BR. Stress-induced hyperglycemia. Crit Care Clin 2001;17(1):107–24.
13. Varon J. Endocrine and metabolic dysfunction syndromes in the critically ill management of the obese critically ill patient. Crit Care Clin 2001;17(1):7.
14. International Diabetes Federation. 56(14):1113–2. Available at: www.idf.org/metabolic_syndrome. Accessed September 22, 2013.
15. Salvatore M, Filion KB, Genest J, et al. The metabolic syndrome and cardiovascular risk: a systematic review and meta analysis. J Am Coll Cardiol 2010;56(14): 1113–32.
16. Karason K, Wallentin I, Larsson B, et al. Effects of obesity and weight loss on left ventricular mass and relative wall thickness: survey and intervention study. BMJ 1997;315(7113):912–6.
17. Marik P, Varon J. The obese patient in the ICU. Chest 1998;113(2):492–8.
18. Vgontzas AN, Tan TL, Bixler EO, et al. Sleep apnea and sleep disruption in obese patients. Arch Intern Med 1994;154:1705–11.
19. Young T, Palta M, Dempsey J, et al. The occurrence of sleep-disordered breathing among middle-aged adults. N Engl J Med 1993;328:1230–5.
20. Punjabi NM, Sorkin JD, Katzel LI, et al. Sleep-disordered breathing and insulin resistance in middle-aged and overweight men. Am J Respir Crit Care Med 2002;165:677–82.
21. Rajala R, Partinen M, Sane T, et al. Obstructive sleep apnea syndrome in morbidly obese patients. J Intern Med 1991;230:125–9.
22. Richman RM, Elliott LM, Burns CM, et al. The prevalence of obstructive sleep apnea in an obese female population. Int J Obes Relat Metab Disord 1994;18: 173–7.
23. Davis G, Patel JA, Gagne DJ. Pulmonary considerations in obesity and the bariatric surgical patient. Med Clin North Am 2007;91:433–42.
24. Frey WC, Pilcher J. Obstructive sleep-related breathing disorders in patients evaluated for bariatric surgery. Obes Surg 2003;13:676–83.
25. Morrell MJ. Residual sleepiness in patients with optimally treated sleep apnea: a case for hypoxia-induced oxidative brain injury. Sleep 2004;27:186–7.
26. O'Keeffe T, Patterson EJ. Evidence supporting routine polysomnography before bariatric surgery. Obes Surg 2004;14:23–6.
27. Van Kralingen KW, de Kanter W, de Groot GH, et al. Assessment of sleep complaints and sleep-disordered breathing in a consecutive series of obese patients. Respiration 1999;66:312–6.
28. McAtee ME. Nursing Care of the Critically Ill Obese Patient. In: El Solh AA, editor. Critical Care Management of the Obese Patient. Oxford, UK: Wiley-Blackwell; 2012.
29. Akinnusi ME, Pineda LA, El Solh AA. Effect of obesity on intensive care morbidity and mortality: a meta-analysis. Crit Care Med 2008;36(1):151–8.
30. Risica PM, Weinstock MA, Rakowski W, et al. Body satisfaction effect on thorough skin self-examination. Am J Prev Med 2008;35(1):68–72.
31. Koenig SM. Pulmonary complications of obesity. Am J Med Sci 2001;321(4): 249–79.

32. Fritts HW Jr, Filler J, Fishman AP, et al. The efficiency of ventilation during voluntary hyperpnea: studies in normal subjects and in dyspneic patients with either chronic pulmonary emphysema or obesity. J Clin Invest 1959;38(8):1339–48.
33. Marik P, Varon J. The obese patient in the ICU. J Chest 1998;113(2):492–8.
34. Chagnac A, Herman M, Zingerman B, et al. Obesity-induced glomerular hyperfiltration: its involvement in the pathogenesis of tubular sodium reabsorption. Nephrol Dial Transplant 2008;23(12):3946–52.
35. Ronco C, Bellomo R, Homel P, et al. Effects of different doses in continuous venovenous haemofiltration on outcomes of acute renal failure: a prospective randomised trial. Lancet 2000;356(9223):26–30.
36. Centers for Disease Control and Prevention: U.S. Department of Health and Human Services. National diabetes fact sheet: general information and national estimates on diabetes in the United States. Available at: http://www.cdc.gov/diabetes/pubs/pdf/ndfs_2007.pdf. Accessed August 14, 2013.
37. Jeffcoate WJ. The incidence of amputation in diabetes. Acta Chir Belg 2005;105(2):140–4.
38. Nelson BV, Van Way CW 3rd. Nutrition in the critically-ill obese patient. Mo Med 2012;109(5):393–6.
39. Garcia Hidalgo L. Dermatological complications of obesity. Am J Clin Dermatol 2002;3(7):497–506.
40. Choban P, Dickerson R, Malone A, et al. A.S.P.E.N. Clinical guidelines: nutrition support of hospitalized adult patients with obesity. JPEN J Parenter Enteral Nutr 2013;37(6):714–44.
41. Blackburn G, Wollner S, Bruce B, et al. Nutrition support in the intensive care unit. Arch Surg 2010;145(6):533–8.
42. Dickerson RN, Boschert KJ, Kudsk KA, et al. Hypocaloric enteral tube feeding in critically ill obese patients. Nutrition 2002;18(3):241–6.
43. Cutts ME, Dowdy RP, Ellersiek MR, et al. Predicting energy needs in ventilator-dependent critically ill patients: effect of adjusting weight for edema or adiposity. Am J Clin Nutr 1997;66:1250–6.

Nutritional Requirements After Bariatric Surgery

Gordana Bosnic, MS, RD, LDN

KEYWORDS

- Bariatric surgery • Postoperative bariatric • Bariatric diet • Postoperative diet stages
- Dumping syndrome • Micronutrient supplementation • Nutrition support

KEY POINTS

- Postoperative nutritional requirements after bariatric surgery vary.
- Bariatric surgeries share common nutritional goals.
- Staged protocol-based meal progression in bariatric patients is recommended after surgery.
- Prevention of dumping syndrome requires dietary modifications to avoid associated symptoms.
- Nutrient intake may be inadequate because of restrictive or nutrient malabsorptive components of bariatric surgeries.
- Adequate fluid intake is important to prevent dehydration.
- Patients may require nutrition support after bariatric surgery.
- Progress toward successful weight loss does not stop with the bariatric surgery.

INTRODUCTION

The nutritional care of the bariatric patient is a fine balance between bariatric diet protocols and individual postoperative dietary tolerances. The role of a registered dietitian (RD) in postoperative bariatric care is to adapt the established bariatric diet protocols to individual tolerances, lifestyles, and nutritional requirements.

MANAGEMENT GOALS

Bariatric surgery diet protocols are surgeon specific and may vary in the progression of diet stages. However, they all share common nutritional goals[1]:

- Maximize weight loss and absorption of nutrients
- Maintain adequate hydration
- Avoid vomiting and dumping syndrome

Conflict of Interest: The author is employed by Sodexo, USA.
Food and Nutrition Department, Winchester Hospital, 41 Highland Avenue, Winchester, MA 01890, USA
E-mail address: gbosnic@winhosp.org

Crit Care Nurs Clin N Am 26 (2014) 255–262
http://dx.doi.org/10.1016/j.ccell.2014.02.002
0899-5885/14/$ – see front matter © 2014 Elsevier Inc. All rights reserved.

The nutritional care after bariatric surgery focuses on adequate energy and nutrient intake to support postoperative tissue healing and preservation of lean body mass during rapid weight loss.[2] The foods and beverages consumed should minimize reflux, early satiety, and dumping syndrome and maximize weight loss and later weight maintenance.[2] Patients should be advised to avoid pregnancy before bariatric surgery and for 12 to 18 months after surgery. Those who become pregnant after bariatric surgery should be counseled and monitored for appropriate weight gain, nutritional supplementation, and for fetal health.[3]

Diet Stages and Progression

A staged protocol-based meal progression in bariatric patients is recommended after surgery. To improve surgical outcomes, patients should receive instructions on their specific bariatric surgery's postoperative diet stages before the surgery.[2] A low-sugar or sugar-free clear liquid diet can usually be initiated within 24 hours[3] after a bariatric procedure and then progressed in accordance with the surgeon's protocol and tolerance. Water is typically the first step toward clear liquids. The clear liquids are usually at room temperature, recommended for 1 to 2 days, and most commonly include diet gelatin, broth, sugar-free popsicles, decaffeinated or herbal teas, artificially sweetened beverages, and in some protocols diluted fruit juices.[2] Bariatric clear liquids exclude sugar, carbonation, caffeine, and alcohol and avoid the use of straws.[1,2]

A low-sugar or sugar-free full liquid diet follows the clear liquid diet. Full liquids commonly include milk (use cautiously with lactose intolerance after bariatric surgery) and milk alternatives, vegetable juice, plain or artificially sweetened yogurt (without fruit pieces), strained cream soups, cream cereals, and sugar-free puddings.[2] Diet progression varies based on surgeon's protocol and patient's tolerance. Most commonly full liquids are recommended for 10 to 14 days[2] and longer on some protocols. Protein supplements should be included to meet the dietary protein needs of the patient.

A pureed diet is typically the diet texture that follows full liquids on the bariatric diet protocol. It consists of foods that have been blended and liquefied and can range from milkshake to mashed potato consistency. Scrambled eggs, egg substitute, flaked fish, pureed meats and meat alternatives, pureed fruits and vegetables, soft cheeses, and hot cereal are often included.[2] Pureed diets are commonly advised for 10 to 14 or more days and protein supplements are continued during this diet stage to supplement protein intake.[2]

Following the pureed diet, patients progress to a bariatric soft diet and remain on this diet stage for the next 14 or more days.[2] It commonly includes ground and chopped tender meats and meat alternatives, canned fruit, soft fresh fruit, canned vegetables, soft cooked vegetables, and grains as tolerated. It is important to keep food moist, especially meat. After 6 to 8 weeks from the surgery, patients typically progress to a regular bariatric diet.[2] During this time patients should transition from 6 small to 3 small meals with scheduled snacks during the day. Patients should chew small bites of food thoroughly and slowly before swallowing. Protein-rich foods should be consumed first during a meal. Protein supplements are continued if patients are unable to meet their protein needs with meals and snacks.

All bariatric diet stages often avoid or delay introduction of[2]:

- Sugar, concentrated sweets
- Carbonated beverages
- Fruit juice (undiluted)

- High-fat foods
- Soft doughy breads, pasta, rice
- Tough, dry, red meat
- Nuts, popcorn, other fibrous food
- Alcohol
- Caffeine

DUMPING SYNDROME

Dumping syndrome can present as a combination of postprandial gastrointestinal, vasomotor, and neuroglycopenic symptoms and occurs in up to 76% of patients after laparoscopic Roux-en-Y gastric bypass (RYGB).[4] It can be early or late, depending on the timing of occurrence of symptoms after a meal. Gastrointestinal symptoms (mostly early dumping) include early satiety, nausea, cramps, and explosive diarrhea.[5] Vasomotor symptoms (both early and late dumping) include sweating, flushing, palpitations, dizziness, and an intense desire to lie down.[5]

Early dumping symptoms occur 10 to 30 minutes after a meal and result from accelerated gastric emptying of hyperosmolar content from the stomach into small bowel. Late dumping occurs 1 to 3 hours after a meal and is a consequence of reactive hypoglycemia resulting from an excessive release of insulin.[5] Rapid delivery of a meal to the small intestine leads to an initial higher concentration of carbohydrates in the proximal small bowel, followed by rapid absorption of glucose into the blood, followed by release of insulin responsible for the subsequent reactive hypoglycemia.[5] To prevent dumping syndrome patient should[1,5]:

- Avoid simple sugars/carbohydrates
- Avoided liquids for at least a half-hour after a meal
- Consume 6 small meals
- Avoid all greasy food, including high-fat starchy food
- Consume adequate fiber when tolerated

NUTRIENTS

Regular follow-ups with an RD are important to facilitate adequate weight loss and manage nutrient intake. Nutrient intake after gastric surgery may be inadequate because of restrictive or nutrient malabsorptive components of the surgeries.[1,6,7] Laparoscopic adjustable gastric banding (LAGB), laparoscopic sleeve gastrectomy (LSG), laparoscopic RYGB, and laparoscopic biliopancreatic diversion (BPD), BPD/duodenal switch (BPD-DS), or related procedures are primary weight loss surgeries.[3]

LAGB consists of placement of an adjustable silicone ring around the upper part of the stomach, creating a small gastric pouch.[8] Injection into or removal of saline from the band's reservoir tightens or loosens the band's internal diameter, thus changing the size of the gastric opening.[4] With the LSG procedure, the stomach is restricted by stapling and dividing it vertically and removing approximately 80% of the greater curvature, leaving a tubular banana-shaped remnant stomach along the lesser curvature.[4] RYGB is the most commonly performed procedure and involves creation of a 10-mL to 30-mL gastric pouch by surgically separating or stapling the stomach across the fundus.[4] Outflow from the pouch is accomplished by performing a narrow (10 mm) gastrojejunostomy. The distal end of the jejunum is then anastomosed 50 to 150 cm below the gastrojejunostomy.[4] The BPD procedure consists of a partial-sleeve gastrectomy with preservation of the pylorus and creation of a Roux limb with a short common channel.[8] The BPD-DS is a variant of the BPD that preserves the first portion of the duodenum.[4]

BPD and BPD-DS are malabsorptive procedures.[6,7] BPD and BPD-DS carry a greater nutritional risk for protein and calorie malnutrition as well as micronutrient deficiencies because of their mainly malabsorptive mechanism of action.[6] LAGB and LSG are mainly restrictive procedures with a neurohormonal component to LSG.[6,7] RYGB has restrictive, malabsorptive, and neurohormonal properties,[6] which means that multiple functional and hormonal changes involved in hunger, food intake, satiety, and glucose metabolism occur after bariatric procedures, resulting in varying weight loss and comorbidity improvement outcomes depending on the procedure. Changes in gut hormones, including ghrelin, glucagonlike peptide-1, and peptide YY, have been associated with the LSG, RYGB, BPD, and BPD-DS procedures.[4]

PROTEIN

Recommendations for protein intake should be individualized. Higher protein intake levels (80–90 g/d) are associated with reduced loss of lean body mass.[3] However, meeting protein needs following the surgery is challenging. Minimal recommended protein intake ranges from 60 g/d to 70 g/d and up to a goal of 1.5 g/kg of ideal body weight.[1,3] BPD/BPD-DS procedures require the amount of protein to be increased by ~30% to allow for malabsorption with an average protein requirement for those patients of ~90 g/d.[2] Patients are encouraged to eat high-protein lean foods before vegetables, fruit, or grains and to distribute protein intake throughout the day in a structured way. Protein supplements are recommended to meet protein needs after surgery. Patients often report that taste and oral tolerance of protein supplements change compared with before surgery. Finding the right protein supplement, choosing a food protein source or texture that can be tolerated, and consuming protein first during a meal are important strategies in achieving the protein intake goal.

CARBOHYDRATES

Although the emphasis is placed on protein intake after surgery, the goal should be to follow the principles of healthy eating, including lean protein, fruits, vegetables, and whole grains.[3,6] Overall daily calorie needs are based on height, weight, age, and activity factors.[1,2]

Sugar and concentrated sweets/simple carbohydrates should be limited after RYGB to avoid dumping syndrome and after any bariatric procedure to reduce caloric intake.[1,3] Fresh fruits and vegetables with fibrous consistency (eg, celery stalks, corn, artichokes) should be avoided or consumed pureed or well cooked[6] because of poor tolerance, especially in the first few months after surgery.

HYDRATION

Adequate fluid intake is important for preventing dehydration and is further complicated with the gastric size limitations after bariatric surgeries. To optimize intake of fluids and to avoid gastrointestinal complications, fluids should not be combined with meals and should be consumed slowly and at least 30 minutes after meals.[3] The amounts vary based on individual needs and generally 1.5 L or more daily provides adequate hydration.[3] Carbonated, caffeinated, caloric, and alcoholic beverages should be avoided or delayed.[2] It is unclear how long an individual should avoid alcoholic beverages. Weight loss and rapid emptying of a gastric pouch contribute to higher blood alcohol content, faster alcohol absorption, and lower metabolic clearance.[3]

MICRONUTRIENTS

After bariatric surgery, patients commonly require micronutrient supplementation in addition to a daily multivitamin with minerals supplement because of the restrictive or malabsorptive nature of the surgical procedures. Basic nutritional daily supplementation recommendations for RYGB and LSG include[3]:

- Two adult multivitamins with minerals (to include iron, folic acid, and thiamine)
- From 1200 to 1500 mg of elemental calcium (in the diet and in the form of citrate supplement in divided doses)
- At least 3000 IU of vitamin D
- Vitamin B_{12} (sublingual, subcutaneous, or intramuscular preparations, or orally if determined to be adequately absorbed) as needed to maintain B_{12} levels in the normal range
- From 45 to 60 mg of iron via multivitamins and additional supplements

BPD/BPD-DS procedures may additionally require fat-soluble vitamin supplementation (vitamins A, E, and K) starting 2 to 4 weeks after surgery.[2] Basic nutritional daily supplementation recommendations for LAGB include[3]:

- One adult multivitamin with minerals including iron, folic acid, and thiamine
- From 1200 to 1500 mg of elemental calcium in the diet and in the form of citrate supplement in divided doses
- At least 3000 IU of vitamin D

Calcium is primarily absorbed in the duodenum and proximal jejunum. It should be supplemented with 1200 to 1500 mg of calcium citrate daily in divided doses.[1,3] Calcium citrate is better absorbed than calcium carbonate, but if patients use calcium carbonate, the recommendation increases to 2000 mg daily. Calcium intake primarily in the form of food has been advocated recently in patients after LAGB because of reports linking calcium supplementation with increased incidence of myocardial infarction risk in women.[3] Vitamin D supplementation should be included with calcium[1] and additional doses should be individualized. Vitamin D supplementation of at least 3000 IU/d is needed in many patients after bariatric surgery.[3]

Iron is primarily absorbed in duodenum and proximal jejunum. Iron deficiency after bariatric surgery can occur because of decreased iron absorption because of less gastric acid being available, poor tolerance of red meat, and menstrual cycles. Patients should wait 2 hours or more after taking an iron-containing supplement to take calcium supplements for optimal absorption.[1,2]

Vitamin B_{12} deficiency can be caused by inadequate contact with intrinsic factor or low intake of vitamin B_{12}–rich foods because of the small size of the gastric pouch.[1] To maintain normal vitamin B_{12} levels, oral crystalline vitamin B_{12} (1000 μg or more daily) or intranasal vitamin B_{12} (500 μg weekly) may be considered.[3] If B_{12} levels cannot be maintained within the normal range with oral or intranasal supplementation, intramuscular or subcutaneous supplementation of 1000 μg/mo or 1000 to 3000 μg every 6 to 12 months is recommended.[3] Low levels of vitamin B_{12} can be seen as soon as 6 months after bariatric surgery, but most often occur more than 1 year after surgery as liver stores are depleted.[2] Vitamin B_{12} deficiency screening should be done routinely at baseline and after surgery and additionally conducted annually for procedures that exclude the lower part of the stomach, such as LSG and RYGB.[3]

Thiamine deficiency after bariatric surgery may manifest as Wernicke-Korsakoff syndrome (WKS) or beriberi.[8] WKS is a combination of mental confusion, ophthalmoplegia, gait ataxia, memory loss, and confabulation. Wet beriberi, also referred to as bariatric beriberi, manifests as a high-output congestive heart failure syndrome characterized by an enlarged heart with normal sinus rhythm and dependent edema.[8] Chronic nausea and vomiting has been associated with thiamine deficiency in patients after bariatric surgery. Thiamine should be included as part of routine multivitamin with minerals supplementation. Screening for thiamine deficiency and additional thiamine supplementation should be considered after surgery in patients with rapid weight loss, protracted vomiting, parenteral nutrition, excessive alcohol use, neuropathy or encephalopathy, or heart failure. Patients with suspected or established severe thiamine deficiency should be treated with intravenous thiamine.[3] Before initiating nutrition support or dextrose-containing solutions, thiamine deficiency should be taken into consideration to prevent WKS.[2] It is recommended that patients with history of bariatric surgery and vomiting receive 100 mg of thiamine with the first bag of dextrose-free intravenous fluid when admitted to an acute care setting such as an emergency department or hospital.[8] Patients with severe thiamine deficiency require higher doses of intravenous thiamine repletion.[3]

Zinc deficiency should be considered in bariatric patients with hair loss, pica, significant dysgeusia, or in male patients with hypogonadism or erectile dysfunction.[3] Patients undergoing a malabsorptive surgical procedure after bariatric surgery should have routine screening for zinc deficiency and should be routinely supplemented following BPD/BPD-DS. Patients being treated for zinc deficiency or using supplemental zinc should receive 1 mg of copper for each 8 to 15 mg of zinc to prevent copper deficiency masked by zinc supplementation.[3]

Copper guidelines for bariatric patients have recently been added, recommending supplementation of 2 mg/d.[3] Copper should be included as part of routine multivitamin with minerals preparation, although some patents may require additional oral treatment or intravenous copper repletion.[3] Screening is not routinely indicated following the surgery, but should be considered in patients with anemia, neutropenia, myeloneuropathy, and impaired wound healing.[3]

Selenium levels should be checked in bariatric patients undergoing a malabsorptive bariatric surgical procedure and presenting with unexplained anemia or fatigue, persistent diarrhea, cardiomyopathy, or metabolic bone disease.[3] Routine selenium screening and supplementation is not recommended at this time.

Vitamin and mineral supplementation should be in chewable or liquid form initially for 3 to 6 months unless inadequate absorption is noted.[2,3]

NUTRITION SUPPORT

After bariatric surgery, patients may require nutrition support because of inability to tolerate oral intake or meet their nutritional needs, or may require surgical procedures including revisions. Nutrition support should be considered in patients after bariatric surgery at high nutritional risk, and severe malnutrition should prompt hospital admission for initiation of nutritional support.[3] Surgeons are sometimes able to place a gastrostomy feeding tube in the remnant stomach of patients after RYGB and the enteral nutrition (EN) support can be administered. Parenteral nutrition (PN) is reserved for patients who cannot meet their nutritional needs with EN. PN should be considered in patients who[3]:

- Are unable to meet their nutritional needs using their gastrointestinal tract for at least 5 to 7 days with noncritical illness

- Are unable to meet their nutritional needs using their gastrointestinal tract for 3 to 7 days with critical illness
- Present with severe protein malnutrition and/or hypoalbuminemia, not responsive to oral or EN protein supplementation

ACHIEVING SUCCESS

Bariatric surgery is a tool to optimize weight loss and minimize comorbidities. Achieving successful weight loss does not stop with the surgery. It begins with the surgery. Patients after bariatric surgery should:

- Adhere to the bariatric diet protocol
- Choose low-fat and low-sugar foods and beverages[6]
- Eat at scheduled times and avoiding grazing[6]
- Regularly follow up with the physician obesity specialist or primary care physician[6]
- Participate in bariatric surgery support groups after discharge from the hospital[3]
- Incorporate moderate aerobic physical activity to include a minimum of 150 minutes per week and a goal of 300 minutes per week, including strength training 2 to 3 times per week[3]
- Continue regular follow-ups with an RD[3]
- Visits with an RD and behavioral therapist any time a patient has difficulty maintaining dietary goals or regaining weight[6]
- Undergo routine screenings for vitamin and mineral deficiencies[3]
- Try to secure a good support system at home[1]

SUMMARY

The postoperative nutritional requirements of a patient after bariatric surgery vary based on the surgical procedure, individual tolerance, and lifestyle. The role of an RD is to adapt the established bariatric diet protocols to individual tolerances, lifestyles, and nutritional requirements. Compliance with the diet protocols as well as regular postoperative screenings for nutrient deficiencies, follow-ups with the bariatric multidisciplinary team, and physical activity can determine the overall success of the bariatric surgery for weight loss.

REFERENCES

1. Academy of Nutrition and Dietetics. Nutrition care manual®. Bariatric surgery. Available at: http://nutritioncaremanual.org/topic.cfm?ncm_category_id=1&lv1=5545&lv2=16927&ncm_toc_id=16927&ncm_heading=Nutrition%20Care. Accessed October 15, 2013.
2. Allied Health Sciences Section Ad Hoc Nutrition Committee, Aills L, Blankenship J, et al. ASMBS allied health nutritional guidelines for the surgical weight loss patient. Surg Obes Relat Dis 2008;4:S73–108.
3. Mechanick J, Youdim A, Jones D, et al. Clinical practice guidelines for the perioperative nutritional, metabolic, and nonsurgical support of the bariatric surgery patient – 2013 update: cosponsored by American Association of Clinical Endocrinologists, The Obesity Society, and American Society for Metabolic & Bariatric Surgery. Surg Obes Relat Dis 2013;9:159–91.
4. Kushner R, Neff L. Surgery for severe obesity. Am J Mens Health 2013;7:255–64.
5. Ukleja A. Dumping syndrome: pathophysiology and treatment. Nutr Clin Pract 2005;20:517–25.

6. Kulick D, Hark L, Deen D. The bariatric surgery patient: a growing role for registered dietitians. J Am Diet Assoc 2010;110:593–9.
7. Snyder-Marlow G, Taylor D, Lenhard J. Nutrition care for patients undergoing laparoscopic sleeve gastrectomy for weight loss. J Am Diet Assoc 2010;110:600–7.
8. Fujioka K, DiBaise J, Martindale RG. Nutrition and metabolic complications after bariatric surgery and their treatment. JPEN J Parenter Enteral Nutr 2011;35:52S–9S.

Bedside Caregivers as Change Agents

Implementation of Early Enteral Nutrition in Critical Care

Miranda K. Kelly, DNP, APRN[a,b,*]

KEYWORDS

- Enteral nutrition • Tube feeding • Evidence-based practice • Change agent
- Critical care • Implementation

KEY POINTS

- Bedside caregivers are in a key position to assess the need for change and implement evidence-based practice at the bedside.
- The Institute of Medicine supports and recommends that nurses be encouraged to collaborate with health care providers to lead change to improve practice environments.
- Early enteral nutrition, within 24 to 48 hours after admission, and use of protocols are recommended by the American Society of Parenteral and Enteral Nutrition guidelines for nutrition support therapy.

INTRODUCTION

Patients in the intensive care unit (ICU) are critically ill yet many do not receive adequate and timely nutritional support. Factors that affect nutritional support are related to institutional system issues, providers, nursing staff, and the patients themselves.[1] Enteral nutrition (EN) is the recommended method of nutritional support and is supported by multiple studies and the 2009 American Society for Parenteral and Enteral Nutrition (ASPEN) guidelines. Despite these recommendations, not all hospitals and providers have embraced the recommendations. Implementation of evidence-based practice can be successful with bedside caregivers as change

Disclosures: The author declares no conflict of interest or financial interests to disclose relating to the content of this article.

[a] Critical Care Units, Memorial Hermann The Woodlands, 9250 Pinecroft Drive, The Woodlands, TX 77380, USA; [b] University of Texas-Health Science Center, 6901 Bertner, Houston, TX 77030, USA

* Critical Care Units, Memorial Hermann The Woodlands, 9250 Pinecroft Drive, The Woodlands, TX 77380.

E-mail address: Mirandak12@sbcglobal.net

agents. An example is a Magnet-recognized community hospital's medical ICU (MICU), which sought to change its practice for EN, with bedside caregivers leading the implementation of an evidence-based protocol.

MODEL FOR CHANGE

To guide the implementation of the EN protocol in the MICU, Larrabee's Model for Change of Evidence-Based Practice was used. Larrabee's model is a revised model that was developed originally by Rosswurm and Larrabee in 1999.[2] Larrabee revised the model based on her own experience, as well as her experience mentoring nurses who used the model.

Larrabee's model for change comprises 6 steps:

1. Assess the need for change in practice
2. Locate the best evidence
3. Critically analyze the evidence
4. Design practice change
5. Implement and evaluate change in practice
6. Integrate and maintain change in practice[2]

Although the steps of the model are progressive, it is not strictly a linear model. Activities in 1 step may prompt activity in another step previously completed. Key aspects of change are identified in **Box 1**. Larrabee's model is used as a format for this article in relation to the practice change project in the MICU.

ASSESS THE NEED FOR CHANGE IN PRACTICE
Development of a Team and Identification of the Clinical Problem

The change agents for the MICU project were bedside caregivers led by the nurse practitioner (NP) and registered dietitian (RD). Bedside caregivers are able to provide information required to identify the need for change and also promote successful implementation. The Institute of Medicine (IOM) recommends that nurses be full partners with other health care professionals in redesigning health care in their report *The Future of Nursing Leading Change, Advancing Health*. The IOM report further

---

Box 1
Key aspects of change in practice

- Develop a team, select a clinical problem, and collect data about the practice
- Review the literature to determine best practice and benchmarks for the change
- Identify an evidence-based project and sets goals
- Complete a thorough literature search to determine sources of evidence and the most appropriate type of project
- Complete a critical analysis of the literature to determine relevance to the project
- Evaluate the practice change to determine feasibility, benefit, and risk
- Design the change, identifying the outcomes and implementation plan
- Pilot, evaluate, and redesign the project
- Integrate and maintain the change

Adapted from Larrabee JH. Nurse to nurse evidence-based practice. New York: McGraw-Hill; 2009. p. 21–35.

recommends that organizations expand nurses' ability to manage collaborative efforts to redesign and improve practice environments.[3] Nurses and all health care providers are encouraged to seek out and implement evidence-based practice (EBP) at the community hospital in which the practice change project was implemented. This support proved to be important in providing the needed support for the EN practice change.

Change agents are the opinion leaders, providing communication, education, and support for the project. An important aspect of that change is obtaining support from all levels of the institution. Change agents for the MICU obtained support from the nurses, providers, nursing and medical directors, and hospital administration before implementation. Nursing and provider champions were identified to support the process change and provide real-time guidance about use of the EN protocol. Change agents provided communication, monitoring, and reinforcement of the EN protocol, providing the support to maintain the implementation of the EN protocol in the MICU. Involvement of all persons affected by the EN protocol was noted to improve the success of the implementation as well as evolvement of the change into the standard of practice for the unit.

Opportunity for improvement in nutritional support for patients in the MICU at the community hospital was first identified by bedside caregivers. Observations during multidisciplinary rounds noted that patients were not receiving adequate nutritional support in a timely manner and there was inconsistency in practice. These observations were based on informal comparison of the RD's recommendations and what the patient was receiving for nutritional support. To determine baseline data for nutritional support, a performance improvement (PI) review was completed, and findings supported the need for implementation of the EN protocol. Review findings noted that 80% of patients received 80% of their recommended goal rate within 48 hours of initiation of EN. These results were obtained from the fluid balance record on the chart, based on the nurses' documented rate of EN each hour. These results are higher than the findings in the literature, in which patients received an average of 45% to 60% of their recommended goal rate.[1,4–6] Despite the positive results, the average time to reach the goal rate was 35 hours and there was a great deal of inconsistency, leaving room for improvement. Development and use of a standardized protocol based on EBP provided the structure for the improvement.

Most patients in the preimplementation group were admitted to the MICU from the emergency center with a respiratory diagnosis. Respiratory disease, such as chronic obstructive pulmonary disease, can affect patients' nutritional status and contribute to loss of strength and function.[7] Patients in the MICU with respiratory distress are often placed on bilevel positive airway pressure (BIPAP) support, a noninvasive mode of respiratory support. This mode of support requires the patient to wear a mask that covers the nose or nose and mouth, limiting oral intake. Patients may require BIPAP for several days in attempts to prevent use of mechanical ventilation. This mode of noninvasive support benefits the patient's respiratory status but contributes to inadequate nutritional support.

Best Practice and Benchmarks for EN

Guidelines such as the ASPEN guidelines are based on EBP and along with protocols are promoted by the IOM. *Crossing the Quality Chasm* is a report from the IOM that identified issues with health care delivery and developed recommendations for improvement.[8] Investigators identified the rapid rate of new medical science and technology and the delay in incorporation into practice. They found that it "takes an average of 17 years for new knowledge generated by randomized controlled trials to be incorporated into practice."[8(p1)] There was delay incorporating the ASPEN guidelines in the MICU, because the guidelines were originally released in 2002.

In 2008, the IOM released another report, *Knowing What Works in Health Care: A Roadmap for the Nation*, which identified techniques for improving health care. The IOM identified that solutions to health care policy issues require one to identify "which diagnostic, treatment, and prevention services really work."[9(p1)] Report investigators recommended developing common language to be used in the development of guidelines and recommendations and encouraged use of systemic reviews to evaluate evidence. Development of clinical practice guidelines promotes effective clinical care, increases use of effective services, and targets populations most likely to benefit.[9] Using the ASPEN guidelines for EN and current evidence are supported by the recommendations from the IOM reports and are the basis for the development of the EN protocol.

Patient safety is an important aspect of the EN protocol and is a priority in the Joint Commission's National Patient Safety Goals.[10] Proactive interventions based on evidence are promoted by the safety goals. Identifying areas of potential error and making clinical and organizational changes have provided direction for the development of an EN protocol and subsequent decrease in complications.[11] Promotion of patient safety in the implementation of EBP changes is a priority.

During multidisciplinary rounds in the MICU, it was noted that patients were not receiving timely and adequate nutritional support. Several factors were identified from these incidental observations that were believed to contribute to patients not receiving adequate nutrition, and they are listed in **Box 2**.

Implementation of the EN protocol in the MICU was based on recommendations from the 2009 ASPEN guidelines, supporting early EN and protocol use.[12] Development of the protocol addressed several areas of concern, including

- Advancement of feeding to goal rate
- Assessment and management of intolerance
- Temporarily discontinuing feedings for tests, procedures, and extubation
- Use of the appropriate size and type of feeding tube

Use of a protocol, including a preprinted order form and algorithm, was identified as an effective tool to improve nutrition in the literature and supported the use in the MICU.[13] The protocol included a preprinted provider's order form for EN and guidelines to initiate EN within 24 hours of the patient not being able to take anything by mouth. The preprinted orders include selection of tube feeding, type of feeding tube, starting rate of feeding, guidelines for increasing to goal rate, and nursing care related to patients receiving tube feedings. An algorithm with guidelines to address gastric residual volume (GRV) (**Fig. 1**), and standardized times for feedings to be temporarily discontinued before procedures was also included. The guidelines addressed the 4 most common reasons noted in the literature for delays, including preparation for a test of procedure, high GRV, hemodynamically unstable patients,

---

Box 2
Factors contributing to inadequate nutrition in the MICU

- Providers' orders for EN rates lower than the recommended rate
- Providers' orders for EN to be held for extended amounts of time before procedures
- Nurses' inconsistent practices of increasing EN to the recommended rate
- Nurses' inconsistent practice of temporarily discontinuing feedings

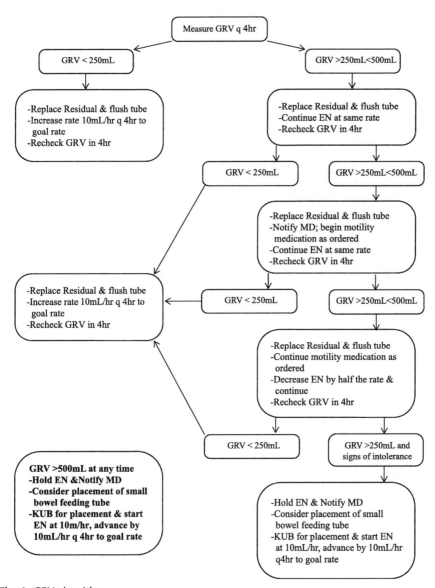

Fig. 1. GRV algorithm.

and nursing care.[1,6,14] With the standardization of nursing care related to EN and use of the guidelines in the protocol, nurses were able to optimize the nutrition that patients receive.

Use of the preprinted order form by providers guided and promoted practice based on evidence and promoted patient safety by providing legible orders. The preprinted order form concept has been incorporated in development of a medical power plan (MPP), with the implementation of computerized provider order entry. The MPP provides the same guidance and links to the evidence that supports the practice. Computerized documentation also promotes safety, because providers place their own orders, so there is no need for interpretation of illegible handwriting.

LOCATING THE BEST EVIDENCE

To determine current EBPs, an extensive review of the literature was completed as part of Larrabee's steps of locating and analyzing the evidence. Ovid, PubMed, and EBSCO search engines were used to search MeSH terms related to EN. The MeSH terms included enteral feeding, tube feeding, EN, protocol, guidelines, guideline adherence, clinician adherence, implementation barriers, and critical care. The terms were searched individually and grouped together to further narrow the search. The MeSH terms that provided the most applicable articles for the protocol were enteral feedings and critical care.

Several research studies supporting implementation of an EN protocol were found during the review of the literature. In a preimplementation and postimplementation comparative analysis of 200 patients, the American College of Chest Physicians found that "utilization of a protocol increased the likelihood that ICU patients would receive EN."[1(p1446)] Despite the results favoring a protocol, patients received only 52% of their daily requirements while receiving EN. The researchers did note a 56% reduction in risk of death, comparing patients with no EN with patients who receive EN, which was clinically significant.

In 1 study, researchers investigated the use of a protocol, as well as an algorithm to prevent aspiration.[15] Researchers compared the preimplementation and postimplementation data and found that implementation of a protocol benefited the patient and that ventilator-associated pneumonias were decreased. However, the researchers did not indicate whether the change was statistically significant.

In another study,[16] researchers compared ICUs that used a protocol with those that did not to determine whether feeding practices improved and if mortality decreased. Researchers reported that more patients received nutritional support and were fed within 24 hours of admission. There was no significant change in patient mortality, but the researchers noted a significant and positive change in practice related to nutrition support.

Individual patient's illnesses can also affect nutritional status. The pathophysiology of the gastrointestinal (GI) tract is interrupted when a patient is critically ill. The motility in the stomach is slowed, pylorus activity is increased, and duodenal activity is disorganized.[17] This change in GI functioning can lead to potential complications with EN, such as aspiration and intolerance. Despite these potential complications, EN is the preferred source for nutritional support, because it contributes to the functional integrity of the GI tract,[18] prevents mucosal atrophy, and preserves gut flora.[19]

Temporary discontinuation of EN has been identified as a contributing factor to patients not receiving their recommended nutritional needs in the literature. Reasons noted for temporary discontinuation included EN being held awaiting tests and procedures; high gastric residuals; and hemodynamically unstable patients.[14,20] Reignier and colleagues[21] reported that not measuring GRV versus measuring GRV was not inferior related to infections acquired in the ICU, mechanical ventilation duration, length of stay, or mortality. Not measuring GRV did improve the delivery of EN by decreasing the amount of time that EN was temporarily discontinued because of high GRV. Inconsistent practice among clinicians compounds this problem and leads to more discontinuations.

CRITICAL ANALYSIS OF THE EVIDENCE

The ASPEN guidelines for EN in the critically ill adult are coauthored by ASPEN and the Society of Critical Care Medicine; both of these groups are leaders in their respective fields.[12] Bankhead and colleagues[11] led a task force of clinical experts that developed general EN practice recommendations supported by ASPEN to determine the validity of the guidelines for the MICU EN project. The Appraisal of Guidelines for Research and Evaluation (AGREE) instrument, which is specific to clinical practice guidelines, was used.[22] The AGREE instrument consists of 23 key items, which are grouped into 6 domains and predict the validity of the guidelines. The findings of this appraisal indicated that the ASPEN guidelines were valid.

The ASPEN guidelines, including recommendations for EN and the critically ill adult, were believed to be relevant to the MICU patient population by the change agents. The standards discussed in the guidelines address route of feeding, timing of feeding, and contraindications for feeding.[11,12] These EN recommendations and guidelines were incorporated in the evidence-based EN protocol for the MICU. The literature and specifically the ASPEN guidelines support the need for protocol use and confirm that there is a gap between EBP and implementation in the clinical setting.[23]

Risks

Potential concerns for successful implementation of changes in practices are identified in the literature. Cahill and colleagues[4] identified barriers related to clinician adherence of clinical practice guidelines, including guideline characteristics, institutional factors, and strategies used for implementation. Brantley[24] identified similar barriers related to guidelines characteristics, strategies of implementation, practitioner attitudes, institutional factors, and patient condition. Identification of barriers and development of implementation strategies should be used by change agents to assist with successful implementation of practice change.

Feasibility

The literature supported that following the ASPEN guidelines and specifically using a protocol would improve nutrition. Protocol use was a feasible option for the MICU, because health care providers were familiar with protocol use. The MICU currently uses protocols for ventilator weaning, blood glucose control, venous thrombosis prophylaxis, and lung volume expansion. The preprinted order form and GRV algorithm were used, having been identified in the literature as effective tools.[13] These practices allowed easier transition, supporting a sustainable standard of care.

Benefits

EN is the preferred route for nutritional support and provides the most benefit based on the evidence. EN contributes to improved wound healing, enhanced immune system function, and improved GI function in general. Parenteral nutrition (PN), the other option for nutritional support, has been associated with gut mucosa atrophy, hyperglycemia, and increased risk for infection.[5] Benefits of EN compared with PN are related to cost, potential complications, and pathophysiology of the GI tract.[17] PN requires placement of a central line, and the cost of PN is higher than EN. Potential complications with EN are related to aspiration and intolerance, whereas potential complications with PN can occur with placement of the line and risk for infection.[17]

Use of the GI tract with EN has been associated with improved outcomes and reduced complications and length of stay.[5] Barr and colleagues[1] noted a decrease in days on mechanical ventilation by 10 days, a shorter ICU length of stay by 8 days, and shorter hospitalizations by 13 days when patients received EN. These findings were clinically significant and provided cost savings to patients and the hospital. McClave and colleagues[18] also noted that improving nutritional support in patients reduced hospital length of stay, decreased infectious morbidity, and decreased cost. PN, which is given intravenously, does not use the GI tract, which contributes to GI atrophy. GI atrophy can promote bacterial translocation and contributes to a higher incidence of infectious complications, which can further contribute to sepsis and decreased survival.[25] Use of the EN protocol promoting best practice can benefit the patient by improving outcomes and the hospital by decreasing costs.

DESIGN OF EN PRACTICE CHANGE

Implementation of EBP changes is typically categorized as PI projects, but it must be ensured that approval from the institutional review board is not required. Development of the EN protocol in the MICU was an interdisciplinary team project, including bedside caregivers as change agents. Disciplines involved in the practice change included the bedside nurses, NP, RD, pharmacist, provider champions, and nursing and medical administrators. Following Larrabee's model, the MICU EN protocol was implemented as a pilot after education was completed for all caregivers. All patients in the MICU, unless excluded, who were unable to take anything by mouth were included, with the identified goal of starting EN within 24 hours. Exclusion criteria included patients who had undergone a surgical procedure, were hemodynamically unstable, or had GI issues such as obstruction, severe diarrhea, or bleeding. Patients on palliative care or hospice care were exclude, because they typically have all orders discontinued. Patients who had an ICU length of stay less than 72 hours or received EN for less than 72 hours were also excluded, because the focus was the first 72 hours of EN.

Outcomes

The objectives for the outcomes of the MICU EN project included the use of the protocol as well as decreasing variability of care affecting patient's nutritional support. Use of the protocol included measuring if the form was used and if the provider and the nurse followed the guidelines. The impact on patients' nutritional support was evaluated by assessing the time that EN was started, the time that patients reached their feeding goal rate, and identifying inconsistencies in management of GRV. All data were obtained from chart review and included a comparison of preimplementation and postimplementation groups, including demographic data.

Demographic data included age, gender, admission source, and admission diagnosis, as shown in **Table 1**. These data points were selected because they were noted to be consistently collected in similar studies of EN implementation.[4,16,25] The items reviewed to evaluate use of the protocol included form use, provider use of recommendations for goal rate, nurse use of guidelines for GRV, and provider and nurse use of guidelines for temporary discontinuation and transition to small bowel feeding tube. Data were collected and percentages for each of the categories were calculated to compare. The overall outcome goal was use of the protocol 50% of the time after implementation.

Evaluation of variability in care was obtained from the documentation in the patient's chart. This variability in care was believed to contribute to amount of EN patients received. Data to evaluate this outcome included time to start feeding, time to feeding goal rate, type of feeding tube, amount of time EN was held for procedures or high GRV, and total calories received per day. Data related to time were compiled, and a mean determined, which was calculated using a t test to determine significance of change. The overall goal was that 80% of patients would reach their feeding goal within 48 hours. The target of 80% was identified after a review of EN studies, in which a caloric intake between 80% and 90% was also used as a target.[1,26,27] Data collection provided an evaluation of the practice change in the MICU and supported further implementation strategies throughout the hospital system.

Table 1
Demographic data from MICU practice change project

Characteristics	Preimplementation (N = 10)	Postimplementation (N = 15)
Gender		
Male	67	56
Female	33	44
Admit source		
Emergency department	80	50
Another hospital	—	—
Extended care	—	13
Floor	—	—
Intermediate care unit	20	37
Admit diagnosis		
Cardiovascular	—	—
Respiratory	100	88
Neurologic	—	—
Gastrointestinal	—	—
Sepsis	—	6
Other	—	6

IMPLEMENTATION AND EVALUATION

Data were collected over 2 3-month periods, one before and one after the implementation of the EN protocol. Data were obtained from charts of patients who received EN. The average age in both groups was 64 years, and most patients were male. Most patients were admitted to the MICU from the emergency department, followed by the intermediate care unit. A respiratory disease process was the admitting diagnosis in most patients.

Medical records of 23 patients receiving EN were reviewed after implementation, with 8 of those patients being excluded. Most patients were excluded because they did not stay in the ICU or receive EN for more than 72 hours, because this was the focus of the practice change project. Other patients were excluded because they were hemodynamically unstable or required surgery. The postimplementation results are based on the 15 remaining patients receiving EN during the 3-month time span of the project.

Practice change outcomes included (1) use of the form and (2) starting EN within 24 hours of cessation of oral nutrition. Although use of the form requires a provider order, both providers and nurses were responsible for initiation. Nurses provided the form for providers and encouraged starting of EN. Use of the EN form in the postimplementation group was 67%, which exceeded the goal of 50%. The goal for starting the EN was within 24 hours and determined from the time that the patient was unable to take anything by mouth until the time that EN was started. In the postimplementation group, the average time was 12 hours, with a standard deviation (SD) of 4.67. This finding was not statistically significant compared with the preimplementation group, which had an average time of 14 hours, with an SD of 14.07. Although there was no statistical difference, there was less variability, as noted by the decrease in SD.

A practice change outcome related to the patients' nutritional support included the percentage of patients who received 80% of the feeding goal rate within 48 hours of initiation of EN. This goal originated from similar studies in the literature,[1,4,24] but the MICU results exceeded the goal, because 100% of patients met the goal. Patients in whom the EN protocol was used reached their goal rate on average 18.5 hours from the start of feeding. **Table 2** compares the mean and median of the patients receiving EN in the preimplementation and postimplementation practice groups for comparison.

All patients in the postimplementation groups combined reached their goal rate on average in 21 hours, with a median of 15 hours. The patients in whom the protocol was used reached 100% of their goal rate on average in 18.5 hours, with a median of 13 hours. Five patients in the postimplementation group reached their goal rate on average in 26.6 hours, despite not having used the protocol order form. This result was believed to be a positive impact of increased focus on nutritional support, providers ordering a goal rate, and nurses advancing to goal rates in a timely manner. Overall, 74% of patients reached their goal rate within 24 hours. In comparison, only 40% of patients in the preimplementation group reached 100% of their goal rate within 24 hours. A 2-sample unequal variance t test with a 2-tail distribution noted a P value of 0.05, which was statistically significant.

Several limitations were identified for the practice change project in the MICU. The project was limited to 1 unit and not representative of all ICUs or acute care areas. Despite this limitation, implementation of EBP changes such as the EN protocol could be easily incorporated into other practices. Nursing documentation limited the collection of data because of incomplete documentation. The lack of documentation, at times covering a 12-hour shift, caused missing data related to intake of EN and limited data reporting.

INTEGRATION AND MAINTENANCE

The final and most important stage of Larrabee's model is that of sustainability. This stage includes confirmation, interpretation, and maintenance of the practice. The nursing staff were very involved with the implementation of the EN practice change and noted that time to feeding goal rate should be 24 hours for all patients. The nursing staff also affected the care of all patients receiving EN, regardless if the protocol order form was used. Nurses advanced feedings to goal rates in a timely manner and consistently treated GRV per the algorithm to improve patients' nutritional support. Nursing staff in the MICU continue to drive the EN protocol, ensuring that EN is ordered within 24 hours of patients' cessation of oral nutrition, GRV guidelines are followed, and patients' nutritional support is optimized.

Communication about the results of the practice change project must include all stakeholders. Results of the MICU practice change project were reported to multiple hospital provider and administrative meetings and, most importantly, to the nurses at their staff meeting. Monitoring of protocol use, continued education, and reinforcement of the protocol have been determined to improve use of guidelines in the literature.[13]

Table 2			
Comparison of time to feeding goal rate in MICU practice change project			
	Preimplementation (N = 10)	Postimplementation: Used Form (N = 10)	Postimplementation: Did Not Use Form (N = 5)
Time to Goal Rate			
Mean (h)	35	18.5	26.6
SD	19.95	12.05	12.30
Median (h)	30	13	23

Box 3
Hot off the press

- 2013 Canadian Clinical Practice Guideline revisions have just been released and ASPEN guidelines are likely to follow
- Web sites with the latest information and EBP guidelines related to nutrition support include
  - American Society for Parenteral and Enteral Nutrition http://www.nutritioncare.org/
  - Critical Care Nutrition criticalcarenutrition.com/
  - Society of Critical Care Medicine http://www.sccm.org/

The MICU and surgical ICU of the project hospital have incorporated the EN protocol into their standard of care. Nutritional support continues to be a focus in daily interdisciplinary rounds, and monitoring of timely nutritional support continues to be a metric for the ICU. Use of the EN protocol has expanded, and it has been successfully implemented in all adult patient care areas of the hospital. The EN protocol framework is being used for implementation of the MPPs, with electronic provider ordering. The practice change project overall has had a positive impact on the patients receiving EN. The goals of the project were all exceeded, as a result of the contribution of to the providers and nursing staff in the MICU.

SUMMARY AND DISCUSSION

Implementation of EBP is the standard of care, yet many guidelines and recommendations are not implemented in a timely manner in the practice setting. Using Larrabee's Model for Change of Evidence-Based Practice bedside caregivers, led by an NP and RD, were able to implement and maintain use of an EN protocol. This protocol provided a standard of care based on the ASPEN guidelines, which continues to affect the nutritional support that patients in the ICUs and adult acute care areas receive. This ICU is 1 example of how bedside caregivers can lead change. Following the IOM's recommendations to encourage nurses to collaborate with other health care providers, bedside caregivers can make an impact, implementing EBP at the bedside. (**Box 3** provides a short list of newly available information in press on the subject.)

REFERENCES

1. Barr J, Hecht M, Flavin K, et al. Outcomes in critically ill patients before and after the implementation of an evidence-based nutritional management protocol. Chest 2004;125:1446–57.
2. Larrabee JH. Nurse to nurse evidence-based practice. New York: McGraw-Hill; 2009.
3. Institute of Medicine. The future of nursing leading change, advancing health. 2010. Available at: http://www.iom.edu/Reports/2010/The-Future-of-Nursing-Leading-Change-Advancing-Health.aspx. Accessed September 3, 2013.
4. Cahill NE, Dhaliwal R, Day AG, et al. Nutrition therapy in the critical care setting: what is "best achievable" practice? An international multicenter observational study. Crit Care Med 2010;38(2):395–401.
5. Heyland DK, Dhaliwal R, Day A, et al. Validation of Canadian clinical practice guidelines for nutrition support in mechanically ventilated, critically ill adult patients: results of a prospective observational study. Crit Care Med 2004;32:2260–5.

6. O'Meara D, Nireles-Cabodevila E, Frame F, et al. Evaluation of delivery of enteral nutrition in critically ill patients receiving mechanical ventilation. Am J Crit Care 2008;17:53–61.
7. Benton MJ, Wagner CL, Alexander JL. Relationship between body mass index, nutrition, strength, and function in elderly individuals with chronic obstructive pulmonary disease. J Cardiopulm Rehabil Prev 2010;30:260–3.
8. Institute of Medicine. Crossing the quality chasm: a new health care system for the 21st century. 2001. Available at: http://iom.edu/Reports/2001/Crossing-the-Quality-Chasm-A-New-Health-System-for-the-21st-Century.aspx. Accessed August 15, 2013.
9. Institute of Medicine. Knowing what works in health care: a roadmap for the nation. 2008. Available at: http://www.iom.edu/reports/2008/knowing-what-works-in-health-care-a-roadmap-for-the-nation.aspx. Accessed August 15, 2013.
10. The Joint Commission. Tubing misconnections–a persistent and potentially deadly occurrence. 2006. In: Sentinel event alert. Available at: http://www.jointcommission.org/sentinelevent/sentineleventalert/sea_36.htm. Accessed August 3, 2013.
11. Bankhead R, Boullata J, Brantley W. Enteral nutrition practice recommendations. JPEN J Parenter Enteral Nutr 2009;33(2):122–67.
12. American Society for Parenteral and Enteral Nutrition (ASPEN) Board of Directors. Clinical guidelines for the use of parenteral and enteral nutrition in adult and pediatric patients. JPEN J Parenter Enteral Nutr 2009;33(3):255–9.
13. Sinuff T, Cook D, Glacomini M, et al. Facilitating clinician adherence to guidelines in the intensive care unit: a multicenter, qualitative study. Crit Care Med 2007; 35(9):2083–9.
14. Elpern EH, Stutz L, Peterson S, et al. Outcomes associated with enteral tube feedings in a medical intensive care unit. Am J Crit Care 2004;13(3):221–7.
15. Bowman A, Greiner JE, Doerschug KC, et al. Implementation of an evidence-based feeding protocol and aspiration risk reduction algorithm. Am J Crit Care 2005;28(4):324–33.
16. Doig GS, Simpson F, Finfer S. Effect of evidence-based feeding guidelines on mortality of critically ill adults. JAMA 2008;300(23):2731–41.
17. Deane A, Chapman MJ, Fraser RJ, et al. Mechanisms underlying feed intolerance in the critically ill: implications for treatment. World J Gastroenterol 2007;13(29): 3909–17.
18. McClave SA, Martindale RG, Vanek VW, et al. Implementation of a nutrition support protocol increases the proportion of mechanically ventilated patients reaching enteral nutrition targets in the adult intensive care unit. JPEN J Parenter Enteral Nutr 2005;29:74–80.
19. Artinian V, DiGiovine B. Effects of early enteral feeding on the outcome of critically ill mechanically ventilated medical patients. Chest 2005;129:960–8.
20. Miller CA, Grossman S, Hindley E, et al. Are enterally fed ICU patients meeting clinical practice guidelines. Nutr Clin Pract 2008;23(6):642–50.
21. Reignier J, Mercier E, Le Gouge A, et al. Effect of not monitoring residual gastric volume on risk of ventilator-associated pneumonia in adults receiving mechanical ventilation and early enteral feeding. JAMA 2013;309(3):249–56.
22. The AGREE Collaboration. Appraisal of guidelines for research and evaluation (AGREE instrument). 2001. Available at: http://www.agreecollaboration.org/. Accessed August 15, 2013.
23. Bourgault AM, Ipe L, Weaver J, et al. Development of evidence-based guidelines and critical care nurses' knowledge of enteral feeding. Crit Care Nurse 2007;27: 17–29.

24. Brantley SL. Implementation of the enteral nutrition practice recommendations. Nutr Clin Pract 2009;24(3):335–43.
25. Khalid I, Doshi P, DiGiovine B. Early enteral nutrition and outcomes of critically ill patients treated with vasopressors and mechanical ventilation. Am J Crit Care 2010;19:261–8.
26. Mackenzie SL, Zygun DA, Whitmore BL, et al. Implementation of a nutrition support protocol increases the proportion of mechanically ventilated patients reaching enteral nutrition targets in the adult intensive care unit. JPEN J Parenter Enteral Nutr 2005;29:74–80.
27. Roberts SR, Kennerly DA, Keane D, et al. Nutrition support in the intensive care unit. Crit care Nurse 2003;23(6):49–57.

Nutrition as Medical Therapy

Dinesh Yogaratnam, PharmD, BCPS[a,*], Melissa A. Miller, PharmD, BCPS[b],
Britney Ross, PharmD, BCPS[c], Michael DiNapoli, PharmD[c]

KEYWORDS

- Selenium • Sepsis • Insulin • Lipid • L-Carnitine • Valproic acid • Toxicity
- Overdose

KEY POINTS

- Intravenous selenium may be a useful therapy for treating severe sepsis; a deadly syndrome for which limited treatment options exist.
- Lipid emulsion therapy has emerged as a viable treatment modality for various toxic drug exposures, including local anesthetic toxicity.
- High-dose insulin therapy has been used successfully to improve cardiac function in patients with acute calcium channel blocker overdose.
- L-Carnitine, which is required for metabolic energy production, has been found to be useful in treating encephalopathy associated with valproic acid toxicity.

INTRODUCTION

Selenium, lipid emulsion, insulin, and L-carnitine are often seen as ingredients in parenteral nutrition formulations. Recent evidence suggests that these agents can also be used to treat various medical conditions that may be encountered in the critical care setting. The indications for these nutritional compounds, the clinical rationale for their use, and the supporting evidence for these therapies are presented in this article.

Funding: None of the authors have funding sources to declare.
Conflicts of Interest: None of the authors have conflicts of interest to declare.
[a] Department of Pharmacy Practice, Massachusetts College of Pharmacy and Health Sciences University, 19 Foster Street, Worcester, MA 01608, USA; [b] Emergency Department, Department of Pharmacy, New York Presbyterian Hospital, Columbia University Medical Center, 622 West 168 Street, New York, NY 10032, USA; [c] Department of Pharmacy, UMass Memorial Medical Center, 55 Lake Avenue North, Worcester, MA 01655, USA
* Corresponding author. Department of Pharmacy, UMass Memorial Medical Center, 119 Belmont Street, Worcester, MA 01605.
E-mail address: dinesh.yogaratnam@umassmemorial.org

SELENIUM FOR SEPSIS

Selenium is an essential nutrient for human health. Selenoproteins are responsible for many of the important physiologic actions of selenium. For example, glutathione peroxidases are a group of antioxidant selenoproteins that protect biomembranes and DNA against damage caused by reactive oxygen species (eg, hydrogen peroxide). Iodothyronine deiodinases, another group of selenoproteins, are responsible for converting thyroxine (T4) to the active thyroid hormone triiodothyronine (T3). Selenoproteins also support the immune system by enhancing the activity and proliferation of T cells and natural killer cells.[1,2]

Deficiency in selenium has been shown to negatively affect health. Increased rates of cancer-associated mortality have been associated in countries where dietary intake of selenium is low. Certain viral infections, including human immunodeficiency virus, similarly may be more likely to lead to clinical deterioration in the setting of low plasma selenium levels.[1,2]

In recent years, there has been a growing body of research showing that high-dose selenium supplementation may have a positive impact on clinical outcomes in sepsis syndromes.[3–5] Although it is not currently known whether the low serum selenium levels observed in sepsis are pathogenic or simply a marker of disease severity, it has been hypothesized that intravenous selenium supplementation, in superphysiologic doses, may provide beneficial antioxidant and antiinflammatory activity that may improve morbidity and mortality from sepsis.[2–5]

Sepsis is defined as the presence of probable infection with systemic manifestations of infection, and severe sepsis is defined as sepsis plus resultant organ dysfunction or tissue hypoperfusion.[6,7] In the United States, severe sepsis accounts for nearly 10% of all intensive care unit admissions, and it is associated with a mortality between 20% and 30%.[7] There is currently no recommended drug therapy that targets the systemic inflammatory response syndrome (SIRS), which is associated with sepsis.[7] An intravenous formulation of selenium, sodium selenite, has recently been investigated as a potential therapeutic option to help to improve clinical outcomes in patients with severe sepsis and septic shock.

Angstwurm and colleagues[4] evaluated the effects of selenium supplementation in patients with SIRS, sepsis, and septic shock in a prospective, randomized, placebo-controlled, multicenter study. This trial enrolled 249 patients, and randomized them to receive 1000 μg of sodium selenite as a 30-minute bolus injection, followed by 1000 μg per day delivered as continuous intravenous infusion for 14 days. Although 28-day mortality did not differ between placebo-treated patients and selenium-treated patients, there were several patients in whom the study protocol was severely violated. Among the 189 patients who received treatment as per protocol, adjuvant selenium was associated with a significant reduction in 28-day mortality compared with placebo (42.4% vs 56.7%; $P = .049$). In a subgroup analysis, a similar mortality benefit in favor of selenium therapy was noted among patients with septic shock, as well as among the most critically ill patients according to Acute Physiology and Chronic Health Evaluation (APACHE) III scores. Serum selenium levels and glutathione peroxidase activity were noted to be in the upper normal range among treated patients and deficient among patients who received placebo.

Manzanares and colleagues[5] performed a prospective, randomized, single-blinded trial of selenium supplementation in 35 patients with SIRS. Within 24 hours of admission to the intensive care unit, patients were randomized to receive intravenous selenium (as sodium selenite) 2000 μg over 2 hours or placebo, which was then followed by a continuous infusion of 1600 μg per day of sodium selenite or placebo for 10 days.

Compared with placebo, patients who received selenium supplementation had a significantly lower incidence of early (ie, ≤5 days) ventilator-associated pneumonia (37.5% vs 6.7%; P = .04) and a greater improvement in severity of illness as measured by the change in Sequential Organ Failure Assessment (SOFA) scores (4.7 vs 7.8; P = .02). Duration of mechanical ventilation, days of antibiotics, hospital and intensive care unit lengths of stay, and mortality were similar between those who received selenium and those who received placebo.

Not all studies of selenium have resulted in positive outcomes.[8,9] Forceville and colleagues[8] performed a prospective, randomized, placebo-controlled, double-blinded, multicenter study of sodium selenite for the treatment of septic shock. In this trial, intravenous sodium selenite was administered as a continuous infusion of 4000 μg on day 1, followed by a continuous infusion of 1000 μg per day for the next 9 days. Unlike the aforementioned studies, clinical benefits of selenium therapy were not observed. Median time to vasopressor withdrawal, median duration of mechanical ventilation, and mortality were similar between patients who received 10 days of sodium selenite infusion and patients who received placebo. Patients in this trial received a similar cumulative dose of selenium as did patients in the trial by Angstwurm and colleagues[4] (approximately 13 mg vs 15 mg, respectively). It has been suggested that that administering sodium selenite as a bolus, rather than as a continuous infusion, as was done in this study, might allow a beneficial pro-oxidant effect in the early stages of sepsis.[10–12] Although this might partially explain why a clinical benefit was not observed in the trial by Forceville and colleagues,[8] this effect remains speculative and needs to be confirmed in a comparative trial.

Several recent meta-analyses have also resulted in discordant results. Alhazzani and colleagues[13] concluded that high-dose selenium therapy may result in improved mortality, whereas Kong and colleagues[14] concluded that there was no clinical benefit for selenium therapy in sepsis. Although these mixed results highlight that the clinical benefit of selenium is not conclusive, they do share 1 promising result: high-dose selenium therapy seems to be safe and well tolerated in the setting of sepsis and septic shock.

Selenium remains a promising therapy for the treatment of sepsis. The largest randomized controlled trial to date, with an estimated enrollment of 1180 patients, was recently completed (ClinicalTrials.gov, NCT00832039). This trial randomized patients with severe sepsis or septic shock to receive placebo or 1000 μg of sodium selenite as a bolus on day 1 followed by 1000 μg per day as a continuous infusion for up to 21 days. The primary outcome is 28-day all-cause mortality. The results of this multicenter study are eagerly awaited.

LIPID RESCUE THERAPY

Lipid emulsion, which is used in parenteral nutrition formulations as a source of fat calories, has been used as an antidote for toxicity caused by local anesthetics, calcium channel blockers (CCBs), and tricyclic antidepressants. These medications are either highly lipophilic drugs (fat soluble) or cause cardiotoxicity when taken in excess. Two proposed mechanisms by which lipid therapy works as an antidote include alterations in metabolic effects and the lipid-sink theory.[15,16] Weinberg and colleagues,[15] using animal models, proposed that cardiovascular toxicity from bupivacaine could be reversed by lipid therapy. Their research suggests that intravenous lipid emulsion may improve contractility of the myocardium through fatty acid oxidation and production of adenosine triphosphate, a process that is by systemic local anesthetic toxicity. Additional studies have explored the theory that, when lipid therapy is used, a lipid sink is created by forming a lipid compartment that lipophilic drugs are drawn into and away from the site of toxicity.[16]

Animal data translated into successful use in humans by way of case reports. The first case reports include successful resuscitation after cardiotoxicity with ropivacaine and bupivacaine.[17,18] In addition to local anesthetics, verapamil, a lipid-soluble and highly cardioselective nondihydropyridine CCB, is particularly dangerous when taken in excess. In 2009, Young and colleagues[19] first reported full recovery with lipid therapy after a patient developed shock caused by verapamil toxicity. The investigators proposed that the success of the lipid therapy was secondary to the lipophilic properties of the drug and creation of the lipid sink. Tricyclic antidepressants, which have both lipophilic and cardiotoxic properties, have both animal and human studies similarly showing benefit of lipid therapy during toxicity.[20,21] Harvey and Cave[22] report successful treatment following an amitriptyline overdose when lipid therapy was added to standard treatment. Following the initiation of lipid therapy, the patient's hemodynamics improved and reduced the QTc and QRS intervals. Amitriptyline levels that were measured before and after lipid therapy increased, yielding to the lipid sink theory. Several other medications, including propranolol (a highly lipophilic β-blocker), atypical antipsychotics (olanzapine and quetiapine), and lamotrigine, have been the subject of case reports involving lipid therapy.[23–25]

Current guidelines recommend using the 20% lipid emulsion at a bolus dose of 1.5 mL/kg followed by an infusion at a rate of 0.25 mL/kg/min for at least 10 minutes.[26] Blood pressure, heart rate, and other available hemodynamic parameters should be monitored for responsiveness. For patients with asystole or pulseless electrical activity, the 1.5 mL/kg bolus may be repeated if the patient does not respond initially. Consider doubling the rate of the infusion to 0.5 mL/kg/min in patients who have not shown a positive hemodynamic response. These guidelines also recommend that lipid infusions should not extend beyond 2 hours; however, recent cases report longer infusion times.[27]

INSULIN AS AN ANTIDOTE

Insulin is a peptide hormone produced and secreted by the pancreatic beta cells in the islets of Langerhans.[28] Insulin is secreted after a meal, during a fasting state, or in response to a glucose load, and reduces blood glucose concentrations by aiding in the uptake and metabolism of glucose by muscle and adipose tissue.[28] Some medications, including CCBs, may inhibit the release of insulin or induce a state of insulin resistance.

CCBs are a common class of medications used to treat hypertension in adults, and include agents in both the dihydropyridine (ie, amlodipine, nifedipine) and nondihydropyridine (ie, diltiazem and verapamil) classes. According to the 2004 annual report of the American Association of Poison Control Centers toxic exposure surveillance system, cardiovascular agents, including CCBs, were involved in 5.6% (n = 46,470) of toxic exposures in adults more than 19 years of age.[29] Cardiovascular agents are also the fifth leading cause of death among toxic medication exposures, with verapamil and diltiazem being the most common CCBs implicated in fatal exposures.[29]

CCBs exert their therapeutic effect by blocking calcium entry into the cardiac muscle cells, smooth muscle cells, and pancreatic beta-islet cells by inhibiting the L-type voltage gated calcium channels.[30] In therapeutic doses, common side effects of CCBs include reflex tachycardia (dihydropyridine class), direct nodal blocking properties resulting in bradycardia (nondihydropyridine class), peripheral edema, and constipation (verapamil). In overdose, CCBs can produce bradycardia, hyperglycemia, and hypotension and shock caused by peripheral vasodilation and negative inotropic effects, specifically caused by verapamil and diltiazem.[31] CCBs also block the beta-islet cells located in the pancreas, thus inhibiting insulin secretion, leading to hyperglycemia, even in therapeutic doses. High-dose insulin therapy with maintenance of normal blood glucose levels, also known as hyperinsulinemia with euglycemia therapy (HIET), has emerged as a viable treatment option for patients presenting with severe CCB overdose.

Treatment of CCB overdose may include decontamination with orogastric lavage, whole-bowel irrigation, and activated charcoal if the patient presents within 1 hour after ingestion.[30] If the patient is hypotensive, supportive care with fluid boluses of 10 to 20 mL per kilogram of body weight and vasopressor agents may be administered.[30] Other treatment strategies may include increasing extracellular calcium with intravenous calcium salts, such as calcium gluconate or calcium chloride, to be used by cardiac muscle and glucagon to increase intracellular cyclic adenosine monophosphate (cAMP).[30,31] In patients with severe overdose, glucagon and calcium do not consistently improve survival or hemodynamic parameters.[30] HIET has become a more widely accepted treatment option as more studies have been published in recent years. Decreased insulin secretion and insulin resistance may develop when toxic ingestions of CCBs occur, and can even occur at therapeutic doses because of the ability of CCBs to bind to and inhibit insulin release from the pancreatic beta-islet cells. When insulin secretion is inhibited, cardiac and smooth muscle cells are unable to use glucose as an energy source. The hypothesis of HIET is that, by administering high doses of insulin and overcoming insulin resistance, the cardiac and smooth muscles are able to use glucose as an energy source and improve contractility and vascular resistance.[31]

Several case reports, case series, retrospective reviews, and prospective observational studies in humans have been published regarding HIET for CCB toxicity.[32–37] In one case report, a 40-year-old woman presented after ingesting one-hundred 10-mg tablets of amlodipine in a suicide attempt. She developed severe hypotension and somnolence requiring intubation. She was started on dopamine and HIET and transferred to the intensive care unit. Twenty-seven days after arrival at the hospital, the patient was discharged to a psychiatric facility.[32] Another case report describes the success of HIET in correcting hypotension in a patient who presented after an intentional overdose of 2.5 g of diltiazem. The patient received 1500 mL of colloid and 500 mL of crystalloid, calcium chloride, 20 mg of glucagon, and dobutamine and norepinephrine infusions with no improvement in his hemodynamic parameters. Only 40 minutes after HIET was started, the patient's blood pressure had improved. Forty-eight hours later, he was able to be weaned off inotropic therapy.[33] In a case series of 12 patients with toxin-induced cardiogenic shock, 4 of which were caused by CCB, Holger and colleagues[34] describe a HIET protocol that includes initial fluid resuscitation with 20 to 40 mL per kilogram of normal saline bolus, intravenous calcium, intravenous dextrose 10% to maintain a blood glucose concentration of greater than 100 mg per deciliter, and an intravenous insulin infusion titrated to clinical response. Serum potassium concentrations were maintained between 3 and 4.5 mmol per liter, and 11 of the 12 patients survived to hospital discharge. In another case series of 7 patients poisoned with CCB, HIET was used and was successful, with 6 of the 7 patients surviving.[35] Overall, HIET for CCB overdose has shown promise as a treatment option.

High-dose insulin therapy used for CCB overdose may seem surprising and excessive to the inexperienced provider who has not seen a HIET protocol previously. The dose of insulin used for CCB overdose is usually 1 unit per kilogram intravenous bolus followed by 0.5 to 1 unit per kilogram per hour intravenous insulin infusion.[30,31] During high-dose insulin therapy, hypoglycemia and hypokalemia may develop. Blood glucose concentrations should be checked every 30 minutes, and 10% dextrose with 0.45% sodium chloride at 80% of the maintenance rate should be initiated when the insulin bolus is administered.[30] Potassium should also be monitored frequently and repleted as needed. The goal of HIET is to maintain a systolic blood pressure greater than 100 mm Hg and a heart rate greater than 50 beats per minute.[30]

In conclusion, insulin is secreted in response to a glucose load that will be used by muscle tissue as a source of energy. Certain medications can inhibit the release of insulin, including CCBs. When CCB toxicity or overdose is suspected, high-dose insulin therapy should be initiated to improve uptake of glucose in the cardiac and smooth muscle cells to be used as energy and to improve contractility and peripheral vasoconstriction. High-dose insulin with euglycemia therapy has been used for CCB toxicity for more than a decade with good results, and should be the mainstay of CCB overdose.

L-CARNITINE FOR VALPROIC ACID TOXICITY

Carnitine is a quaternary amine synthesized from the amino acids lysine and methionine.[38] Two enantiomers exist, but only levocarnitine (L-carnitine) has biological activity.[39] Endogenous production of carnitine accounts for approximately 25% of total body stores and occurs in various organs including the liver, heart, brain, skeletal muscle, and kidney. About 75% of carnitine comes from dietary intake, primarily from red meat and dairy products.[40,41]

Carnitine facilitates the production of acetyl coenzyme A (CoA), which subsequently enters the Krebs cycle to aid in energy production. Carnitine also helps to maintain the ratio of acetylated CoA to free CoA within mitochondria. This function is important because failure to sustain this ratio can result in impaired energy production and can allow accumulation of acyl CoA compounds.[38,39]

L-Carnitine is commercially available as a tablet, capsule, oral solution, and parenteral solution for intravenous and intramuscular administration.[41] Carnitine is considered safe and well tolerated.[41,42] Rare, but serious, side effects including hypertension, hypotension, tachyarrhythmias, chest pain, headache, hypercalcemia, anemia, and seizures have been reported. These effects have mostly occurred in patients on chronic hemodialysis.[42,43]

Valproic acid (VPA) is a drug used in the treatment of generalized and focal seizures, panic disorder, bipolar disorder, migraine prophylaxis, trigeminal neuralgia, and other neuropathic pain.[40,41] The exact mechanism of action of VPA is unknown. It is thought to increase levels of gamma-aminobutyric acid in the central nervous system (CNS), suppress N-methyl-D-aspartate activity, and have a direct effect on neuronal membranes by altering sodium and potassium conductance.[38] Serious side effects can be seen during acute overdose of VPA, including CNS depression, coma, cerebral edema, hepatotoxicity, hyperammonemic encephalopathy, hypotension, pancreatitis, coagulopathy, bone marrow suppression, and metabolic acidosis.[44]

VPA is extensively metabolized in the liver. Because it possesses a chemical structure akin to short-chain fatty acids, VPA serves as a substrate in the fatty acid oxidation pathway. It needs to be transported into mitochondria via a carnitine shuttle, which is the same pathway used by long chain fatty acids. Approximately 17% of VPA is metabolized via oxidation. A by-product of this, 2-propyl-4-pentanoic acid, has been associated with the development of cerebral edema, hepatotoxicity, and hyperammonemic encephalopathy.[44]

Carnitine deficiency has been associated with VPA therapy, especially during chronic administration or with high doses, as in an acute ingestion. The cause of carnitine deficiency is not completely understood, but it is thought to be the result of numerous synergistic metabolic pathways. First, VPA can alter absorption of carnitine from food, which is a main source of carnitine intake. Second, it can decrease the biosynthesis of carnitine from the liver and kidneys by interfering with gamma-butyrobetaine hydroxylase, which is an enzyme responsible for endogenous production. Third, VPA can decrease the reabsorption of carnitine from the kidneys. Fourth, VPA combines with carnitine to form valproylcarnitine, which is excreted in the urine. Before excretion, valproylcarnitine inhibits the carnitine transporter, decreasing the transport of carnitine into the cell and mitochondria.[44,45]

Carnitine depletion alters oxidative metabolism, resulting in an increased production of toxic metabolites and leading to the myriad of symptoms discussed earlier during acute overdose.[44,46] Patients at increased risk of developing carnitine deficiency include children less than 24 months of age, those with concomitant neurologic or metabolic disorders, those with hepatic or renal failure, or those who use multiple anticonvulsants.[47]

In addition to decreasing carnitine stores, it is well described that VPA can increase ammonia levels.[48–50] The prevalence of hyperammonemia is reported to be between 50% and 70% in patients on VPA, although about half of these patients remain asymptomatic.[48] Hyperammonemia can develop despite normal liver function tests, so its cause is likely independent of hepatotoxicity.[41] Hyperammonemia can lead to significant encephalopathy, cerebral edema, altered mental status, vomiting, and increase in seizure frequency. Risk factors for the development of hyperammonemia include congenital defects of the urea cycle, being on multiple anticonvulsants, eating a protein-rich diet, liver dysfunction, and hypercatabolic states.[51]

It has been postulated that L-carnitine supplementation could attenuate or correct the effects of carnitine deficiency, hyperammonemic encephalopathy, and hepatotoxicity seen during acute VPA overdose. Administration of exogenous L-carnitine normalizes oxidative metabolism in mitochondrial cells of the liver, thus preventing buildup of toxic metabolites.[49,52]

Although quality evidence is limited and mainly based on case reports, carnitine supplementation has been shown to reverse metabolic abnormalities and quicken the resolution of hyperammonemia. Ohtani and colleagues[53] showed that administration of oral carnitine in patients on VPA reduced serum ammonia levels in all 14 patients as the plasma carnitine concentrations normalized. However, restoring ammonia levels has not been shown to hasten the recovery of consciousness. Hantson and colleagues[54] reported a case of a 47-year-old man on VPA who developed severe hyperammonemic encephalopathy. After L-carnitine supplementation, serum ammonia levels returned to normal but the patient remained comatose for 3 weeks. Bohan and colleagues[55] retrospectively analyzed 92 patients on VPA with acute, symptomatic, hepatic dysfunction to determine the effect of L-carnitine on hepatic survival. L-Carnitine treatment was associated with an improvement in survival (48%) compared with aggressive supportive care (10%) ($P<.001$). Hepatic survival was most notable in patients diagnosed within 5 days of ingestion and who were treated with intravenous rather than enteral therapy.

L-Carnitine is generally considered safe and well tolerated, although there are a limited number of studies assessing its safety profile. LoVecchio and colleagues[56] reviewed adverse effects of L-carnitine in patients with acute VPA ingestion over a 3-year period. They found no reported adverse events in the 251 patients who received the drug. However, an important limitation of this study is that the investigators only examined anaphylaxis and hypotension as adverse events. Furthermore, the doses of L-carnitine that were administered were not reported and no statistical analysis of the data was performed. No cases of allergic reactions or other severe reactions have been documented with carnitine administration in patients with acute VPA overdose.[56]

Optimal dosing regimens and treatment durations of L-carnitine in VPA poisoning have yet to be determined. Established dosing ranges exist for L-carnitine supplementation for use in chronic hemodialysis, cancer-related fatigue, and prevention of hepatotoxicity with chronic VPA use, but applying these recommendations to patients with acute VPA poisoning is inappropriate. The US Food and Drug Administration approved labeling is for short-term and long-term treatment of patients with an inborn error of metabolism resulting in secondary carnitine deficiency. There is no mention of dosing recommendations during acute ingestions. Given the CNS depression of patients presenting with severe VPA toxicity coupled with the low bioavailability of oral L-carnitine, intravenous administration is preferred. In addition, patients treated with intravenous L-carnitine have improved outcomes compared with those given enteral administration.[55] Numerous dosing strategies have been used. Most references recommend a loading dose of 50 to 100 mg per kilogram body weight.[49,52,57] Maintenance doses are required for ongoing and delayed absorption. Maintenance dosing has ranged from 15 to 100 mg per kilogram per day with frequencies varying from every 4 hours to daily dosing.[55,57] The Pediatric Neurology Consensus Conference in 1996 and other sources have recommended giving 50 to 100 mg per kilogram per day during VPA poisoning and in VPA-induced hepatotoxicity.[47] One recent study recommends maintenance dosing as 50 mg per kilogram (maximum 3 g per dose) every 8 hours.[57] Furthermore, the Pediatric Neurology Advisory Committee recommends 150 to 500 mg per kilogram per day (maximum 3 g per day) as rescue therapy for VPA-induced hepatotoxicity.[58] Duration of therapy has not been defined, but most literature reports using L-carnitine for 3 to 4 days and suggests treating until resolution of clinical symptoms.[49,52] Doses can be administered as an intravenous bolus over 2 to 3 minutes or by continuous infusion over 30 minutes.[42]

High-quality evidence surrounding the use of L-carnitine in patients with acute VPA toxicity is scarce. However, given the pathophysiology of VPA toxicity and the lack of reported adverse events associated with administration of L-carnitine, its use in this setting remains a reasonable option. Most published evidence recommends using L-carnitine in patients with acute VPA overdose or VPA-induced hepatotoxicity and hyperammonemia. Note that reported evidence using L-carnitine in this clinical scenario introduces publication bias, because unsuccessful case reports are less likely to be published. In addition, optimal dosing regimens, duration of therapy, and safety using L-carnitine during acute VPA toxicity are not established. To do so, further prospective studies including larger patient populations are needed.

SUMMARY

Critical care nurses may typically notice selenium, lipid emulsion, insulin, and L-carnitine as ingredients in parenteral nutrition, but these agents can also be used to treat various medical conditions. By being familiar with the clinical rational, as well as the dosing and side effect profile for these agents, the critical care nurse can aptly prepared to provide optimal care for patients who receive these therapies.

REFERENCES

1. Rayman MP. Selenium and human health. Lancet 2012;379:1256–68.

2. Rayman MP. The importance of selenium to human health. Lancet 2000;356: 233–41.
3. Andrews PJ, Avenell A, Noble DW, et al. Randomised trial of glutamine, selenium, or both, to supplement parenteral nutrition for critically ill patients. BMJ 2011;342:d1542.
4. Angstwurm MW, Engelmann L, Zimmermann T, et al. Selenium in intensive care (SIC): results of a prospective randomized, placebo-controlled, multiple-center study in patients with severe systemic inflammatory response syndrome, sepsis, and septic shock. Crit Care Med 2007;35(1):118–26.
5. Manzanares W, Biestro A, Torre MH, et al. High dose selenium reduces ventilator-associated pneumonia and illness severity in critically ill patients with systemic inflammation. Intensive Care Med 2011;37:1120–7.
6. Angus DC, van der Poll T. Severe sepsis and septic shock. N Engl J Med 2013; 369:840–51.
7. Dellinger RP, Levy MM, Rhodes A, et al. Surviving sepsis campaign: international guidelines for management of severe sepsis and septic shock: 2012. Crit Care Med 2013;41(2):580–637.
8. Forceville X, Laviolle B, Annane D, et al. Effects of high dose selenium, as sodium selenite, in septic shock: a placebo-controlled, randomized, double-blind phase II study. Crit Care 2007;11(4):R73.
9. Heyland D, Muscedere J, Wischmeyer PE, et al. A randomized trial of glutamine and antioxidants in critically ill patients. N Engl J Med 2013;368:1489–97.
10. Forceville X. The effect of selenium therapy on mortality in patients with sepsis syndrome: simple selenium supplementation or real $(5H_2O)\bullet Na_2SeO_3$ pharmacological effect? Crit Care Med 2013;41(6):1591–2.
11. Heyland DK. Selenium supplementation in critically ill patients: can too much of a good thing be a bad thing? Crit Care 2007;11:153.
12. Wang Z, Forceville X, Van Antwerpen P, et al. A large bolus injection, but not continuous infusion of sodium selenite improves outcome in peritonitis. Shock 2009;32(2):140–6.
13. Alhazzani W, Jacobi J, Sindi A, et al. The effect of selenium therapy on mortality in patients with sepsis syndrome: a systemic review and meta-analysis of randomized controlled trials. Crit Care Med 2013;41(6):1555–64.
14. Kong Z, Wang F, Ji S, et al. Selenium supplementation for sepsis: a meta-analysis of randomized controlled trials. Am J Emerg Med 2013;31(8):1170–5.
15. Weinberg GL, VadeBoncouer T, Ramaraju GA, et al. Pretreatment or resuscitation with a lipid infusion shifts the dose-response to bupivacaine-induced asystole in rats. Anesthesiology 1998;88:1071–5.
16. Weinberg GL, Ripper R, Murphy P, et al. Lipid infusion accelerates removal of bupivacaine and recovery from bupivacaine toxicity in the isolated rat heart. Reg Anesth Pain Med 2006;31:296–303.
17. Rosenblatt MA, Abel M, Fischer GW, et al. Successful use of a 20% lipid emulsion to resuscitate a patient after a presumed bupivacaine-related cardiac arrest. Anesthesiology 2006;105:217–8.
18. Litz RJ, Popp M, Steher SN, et al. Successful resuscitation of a patient with ropivacaine-induced asystole after axillary plexus block using lipid infusion. Anesthesiology 2006;61:800–1.
19. Young AC, Velez LI, Kleinschmidt KC. Intravenous fat emulsion therapy for intentional sustained-release verapamil overdose. Resuscitation 2009;80:591–3.
20. Harvey M, Cave G. Intralipid outperforms sodium bicarbonate in a rabbit model of clomipramine toxicity. Ann Emerg Med 2007;49:178–85.

21. Blaber MS, Khan JN, Brebner JA, et al. Lipid rescue for tricyclic antidepressant cardiotoxicity. Emerg Med 2012;43:465–7.
22. Harvery M, Cave G. Case report: successful lipid resuscitation in multi-drug overdose with predominant tricyclic antidepressant toxidrome. Int J Emerg Med 2012;5:1–5.
23. Jovic-Stosic J, Gligic B, Putic V, et al. Severe propranolol and ethanol overdose with wide complex tachycardia treated with intravenous lipid emulsion: a case report. Clin Toxicol (Phila) 2011;49:426–30.
24. Finn SD, Uncles DR, Willers J, et al. Early treatment of a quetiapine and sertraline overdose with intralipid. Anaesthesia 2009;64:191–4.
25. Castanares-Zapatero D, Wittebole X, Huberlant V, et al. Lipid emulsion as rescue therapy in lamotrigine overdose. J Emerg Med 2012;42:48–51.
26. American College of Medical Toxicology. ACMT position statement: interim guidance for the use of lipid rescue therapy. J Med Toxicol 2011;7:81–2.
27. Bologa C, Lionte C, Coman A, et al. Lipid emulsion therapy in cardiodepressive syndrome after diltiazem overdose – case report. Am J Emerg Med 2013;31:1154.
28. Powers AC, D'Alessio D, Powers AC. Chapter 43. Endocrine pancreas and pharmacotherapy of diabetes mellitus and hypoglycemia. In: Brunton LL, Chabner BA, Knollmann BC, et al, editors. Goodman & Gilman's the pharmacological basis of therapeutics. 12th edition. New York: McGraw-Hill; 2011. http://accesspharmacy.mhmedical.com/content.aspx?bookid=374&Sectionid=41266252. Accessed September 5, 2013.
29. Watson WA, Litovitz TL, Rodgers GC Jr, et al. 2004 Annual report of the American Association of poison control centers toxic exposure surveillance system. Am J Emerg Med 2005;23:589–666.
30. Shepherd G. Treatment of poisoning caused by β-adrenergic and calcium channel blockers. Am J Health Syst Pharm 2006;63:1828–35.
31. Lheureux PE, Zahir S, Gris M, et al. Bench-to-bedside review: hyperinsulinemia/euglycemia therapy in the management of overdose of calcium-channel blockers. Crit Care 2006;10(3):212.
32. Harris NS. Case 24-2006: a 40-year-old woman with hypotension after an overdose of amlodipine. N Engl J Med 2006;355:602–11.
33. Abeysinghe N, Aston J, Polouse S. Diltiazem overdose: a role for high-dose insulin. Emerg Med J 2010;27:802–3.
34. Holger JS, Stellpflug SJ, Cole JB, et al. High-dose insulin: a consecutive case series in toxin-induced cardiogenic shock. Clin Toxicol 2011;49:653–8.
35. Engebretsen KM, Kaczmarek K, Morgan J, et al. High-dose insulin therapy in beta-blocker and calcium-channel blocker poisoning. Clin Toxicol 2011;49:277–83.
36. Green SL, Gawarammana I, Wood DM, et al. Relative safety of hyperinsulinemia/euglycemia therapy in the management of calcium channel blocker overdose: a prospective observational study. Intensive Care Med 2007;33:2019–24.
37. Shepherd G, Klein-Schwartz W. High-dose insulin therapy for calcium-channel blocker overdose. Ann Pharmacother 2005;39:923–30.
38. Katiyar A, Aaron C. The use of carnitine for the management of acute valproic acid toxicity. J Med Toxicol 2007;3(3):129–38.
39. Hathcock J, Shao A. Risk assessment for carnitine. Regul Toxicol Pharmacol 2006;46(1):23–8.
40. Flomenbaum NE, Goldfrank LR, Hoffman RS, et al. Goldfrank's toxicological emergencies. 8th edition. Columbus, OH: McGraw-Hill Companies, Inc; 2006.

41. Lheureux P, Hantson P. Carnitine in the treatment of valproic acid-induced toxicity. Clin Toxicol 2009;47:101–11.
42. Levocarnitine [package insert]. Gaithersburg, MD: Sigma-Tau Pharmaceuticals, Inc. 2004.
43. Mock C, Schwetschenau K. Levocarnitine for valproic-acid-induced hyperammonemic encephalopathy. Am J Health Syst Pharm 2012;69:35–9.
44. Lheureux PE, Penaloza A, Zahir S, et al. Carnitine in the treatment of valproic acid-induced toxicity – what is the evidence? Crit Care Med 2005;9(5):431–40.
45. Stadler DD, Bale JF Jr, Chenard CA, et al. Effect of long-term valproic acid administration on the efficiency of carnitine reabsorption in humans. Metabolism 1999;48(1):74–9.
46. Sztajnkrycer MD. Valproic acid toxicity: overview and management. J Toxicol Clin Toxicol 2002;40(6):789–801.
47. DeVivo DC, Bohan TP, Coulter DL, et al. L-carnitine supplementation in childhood epilepsy: current perspectives. Epilepsia 1998;39(11):1216–25.
48. Murphy JV, Groover RV, Hodge C. Hepatotoxic effects in a child receiving valproate and carnitine. J Pediatr 1993;123:318–20.
49. Ishikura H, Matsui N, Matsubara M, et al. Valproic acid overdose and L-carnitine therapy. J Anal Toxicol 1996;20:55–8.
50. Collins RM Jr, Zielke HR, Woody RC. Valproate increases glutaminase and decreases glutamine synthetase activities in primary cultures of rat brain astrocytes. J Neurochem 1994;62:1137–43.
51. Warter JM, Imler M, Marescaux C, et al. Sodium valproate-induced hyperammonemia in the rat: role of the kidney. Eur J Pharmacol 1983;87:177–82.
52. Murakami K, Sugimoto T, Woo M, et al. Effect of L-carnitine supplementation on acute valproate intoxication. Epilepsia 1996;37(7):687–9.
53. Ohtani Y, Endo F, Matsuda I. Carnitine deficiency and hyperammonemia associated with valproic acid therapy. J Pediatr 1982;101(5):782–5.
54. Hantson P, Grandin C, Duprez T, et al. Comparison of clinical, magnetic resonance and evoked potentials data in a case of valproic-acid-related hyperammonemic coma. Eur Radiol 2005;15:59–64.
55. Bohan TP, Helton E, McDonald I, et al. Effect of L-carnitine treatment for valproate-induced hepatotoxicity. Neurology 2001;56:1405–9.
56. LoVecchio F, Shriki J, Samaddar R. L-carnitine was safely administered in the setting of valproate toxicity. Am J Emerg Med 2005;23(3):321–2.
57. Perrott J, Murphy N, Zed P. L-carnitine for acute valproic acid overdose: a systematic review of published cases. Ann Pharmacother 2010;44:1287–93.
58. Raskind JY, El-Chaar GM. The role of carnitine supplementation during valproic acid therapy. Ann Pharmacother 2000;34(5):630–8.

Index

Note: Page numbers of article titles are in **boldface** type.

Crit Care Nurs Clin N Am 26 (2014) 289–295
http://dx.doi.org/10.1016/S0899-5885(14)00020-3
0899-5885/14/$ – see front matter © 2014 Elsevier Inc. All rights reserved.

ccnursing.theclinics.com

Printed and bound by CPI Group (UK) Ltd, Croydon, CR0 4YY

03/10/2024

01040489-0012